Men's Health

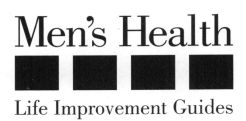

Life Improvement Guides

Symptom Solver

Understanding—And
Treating—The Most Common
Male Health Concerns

by Alisa Bauman, Brian Paul Kaufman
and the Editors of **Men'sHealth** Books

Rodale Press, Inc.
Emmaus, Pennsylvania

Copyright © 1997 by Rodale Press, Inc.

Cover photograph copyright © l996 by Walter Smith
Illustrations copyright © 1996 by Alan Baseden; Barbara Friedman; John A. Nyquist, M.S., CMI

Other titles in the *Men's Health Life Improvement Guides* series:
  Sex Secrets
  Food Smart
  Powerfully Fit
  Fight Fat

Library of Congress Cataloging-in-Publication Data

Bauman, Alisa.
    Symptom solver : understanding—and treating—the most common male
health concerns / by Alisa Bauman, Brian Paul Kaufman and the editors of
Men's Health Books.
        p.   cm.—(Men's health life improvement guides)
    Includes index.
    ISBN 0–87596–357–9 paperback
1. Symptomatology—Popular works. 2. Men—Diseases—Diagnosis.
3. Men—Health and hygiene. I. Kaufman, Brian, 1961– .
II. Men's Health Books.   III. Title.   IV. Series.
RC69.B38   1996
616'.047'081—dc20   96–22076

Distributed in the book trade by St. Martin's Press

2   4   6   8   10   9   7   5   3   1   paperback

—— OUR PURPOSE ——
*"We inspire and enable people to improve
their lives and the world around them."*

Symptom Solver Editorial Staff

Senior Managing Editor: **Neil Wertheimer**

Senior Editors: **Jack Croft, Matthew Hoffman**

Writers: **Alisa Bauman, Brian Paul Kaufman**

Associate Art Director: **Faith Hague**

Series Designer: **John Herr**

Book Designer: **David Q. Pryor**

Cover Designer: **Charles Beasley**

Cover Photographer: **Walter Smith**

Photo Editor: **Susan Pollack**

Illustrators: **Alan Baseden, Barbara Friedman, John A. Nyquist**

Studio Manager: **Joe Golden**

Layout Artist: **Mary Brundage**

Technical Artist: **Thomas P. Aczel**

Researchers and Fact-Checkers: **Elizabeth A. Brown, Raymond M. Di Cecco, Jane Unger Hahn, Sally A. Reith**

Copy Editor: **David R. Umla**

Production Manager: **Helen Clogston**

Manufacturing Coordinator: **Melinda B. Rizzo**

Office Staff: **Roberta Mulliner, Julie Kehs, Bernadette Sauerwine, Mary Lou Stephen**

Rodale Health and Fitness Books

Vice-President and Editorial Director: **Debora T. Yost**

Art Director: **Jane Colby Knutila**

Research Manager: **Ann Gossy Yermish**

Copy Manager: **Lisa D. Andruscavage**

Photo Credits

Page 138, left: **Walter H. Hodge/Peter Arnold, Inc.**

Page 138, center: **Ed Reschke/Peter Arnold, Inc.**

Page 138, right: **Rob Cardillo**

Page 142: **John Abbott Studio**

Page 144: **Jesse Frohman**

Page 146: **Victor Sailor/Photo Run**

Page 148: **Joey Walker**

Back flap: **Everett Collection, Inc.**

Contents

Introduction   **vi**

Part One
Body Talk
Listen to Your Body   **2**
When Germs Invade   **4**
When Your Body Overeacts   **10**
When You Skip Regular Maintenance   **12**
Choosing Your Doctor   **18**
When to See Your Doctor   **26**

Part Two
Head
Bad Breath   **32**
Bleeding Gums   **33**
Canker Sores   **34**
Chapped Lips   **35**
Coughing   **36**
Dizziness   **37**
Ear Pain   **38**
Eye Discomfort   **39**
Fever   **40**
Forgetfulness   **41**
Hair Loss   **42**
Headaches: Tension-Type   **44**
Headaches: Migraine   **46**
Headaches: Cluster   **48**

Jaw Pain   **49**
Nosebleed   **50**
Runny and/or Stuffy Nose   **52**
Sneezing   **54**
Snoring   **55**
Sore Throat   **57**
Swollen Glands   **58**
Toothache   **59**
Vision Problems   **60**

Part Three
Lungs and Heart
Breathing Problems   **62**
Chest Pain   **64**
Heartbeat Irregularities   **67**

Part Four
Stomach and Digestive System
Anal Ailments   **70**
Belching   **71**
Constipation   **72**
Diarrhea   **73**
Gas   **74**
Heartburn   **75**
Incontinence   **77**
Nausea/Vomiting   **79**

Part Five
Sexual Organs
Impotence   **82**

Low Sex Drive   **88**
Premature Ejaculation   **91**
Semen Problems   **92**
Testicular Lumps   **94**
Urination Problems   **96**

Part Six
Arms, Legs and Back

Ankle Pain   **100**
Arm Pain   **103**
Back Pain   **104**
Elbow Pain   **109**
Knee Pain   **111**
Leg Pain   **115**
Muscle Cramps   **117**
Neck Pain   **118**
Shoulder Pain   **120**
Wrist Pain   **122**

Part Seven
Skin

Acne   **126**
Athlete's Foot and Jock Itch   **128**
Body Odor   **130**
Bruises   **132**
Cold Sores   **133**
Dandruff   **134**
Itchy Skin   **135**
Moles   **136**
Rashes   **137**

Unwanted Hair Growth   **139**
Warts   **140**

Part Eight
Real-Life Scenarios

Quest for the Best
Charles M. Harper,   **142**
Former Chairman and
Chief Executive Officer,
RJR Nabisco

Michael Olajidé, Jr.,   **144**
Former World
Middleweight Contender

Mark Conover,   **146**
Olympic Marathoner

Bob Beamon,   **148**
Olympic Gold Medalist

You Can Do It!
Fear Goes Up in Smoke   **150**
Greg Hrabar,
Toms River, New Jersey

Coming to Grips with Cancer   **152**
Joe Dvorak,
South Barrington, Illinois

Back from the Brink   **154**
Charlie Walker,
New Castle, Delaware

A Happy Ending   **156**
John Trout,
Bethlehem, Pennsylvania

Road Map to Health
The Tests of Time   **158**

Index   **164**

Introduction

Managing Your Health

You hear a lot of talk these days about managed health care. Mostly, it's about big corporations who have managed to find a way to charge you more money for less coverage.

Still, it's a concept worth exploring on a personal level: Who's going to manage *your* health care? Don't worry. It's not a trick question. There's really only one correct answer: *You.* Because if you don't, somebody else will. Maybe an emergency room doctor that you've never met before in your life. Or a faceless insurance conglomerate based in some distant state.

The only way you can get the health care that you need—and that you deserve—is to manage your health the way that you would manage a business. Take on the responsibilities that you are qualified to handle and hire the best professionals that you can find to deal with matters outside your expertise.

Consider this your management handbook. We approached *Symptom Solver* making two basic assumptions. The first is that men absolutely hate to go to the doctor, so they want practical information on what they can do to take care of minor health problems themselves. The second is that when it is necessary to go to the doctor, guys want straightforward answers—not medical double-talk—and the appropriate level of treatment.

Symptom Solver will arm you with the knowledge that you need to accomplish both of those goals. You'll find a wide range of quick cures for everything from acne to warts; from athlete's foot to unwanted and embarrassing hair growth. We also offer tips and techniques to relieve more serious problems such as back pain, impotence and joint pain. And when you do need to see a doctor, we'll help you establish the kind of professional relationship that should exist between a man and his physician—one in which you're the boss. Because to put it bluntly, your doctor works for you.

That means that you are entitled to the same level of respect and responsiveness that you would expect from any other professional you hire for his expertise, whether it's an accountant, a lawyer, a management consultant or an automobile mechanic.

If some inconsiderate cretin dents your car in a mall parking lot, what would you do? If it's a minor scratch, you'd probably fix it yourself. If it's a serious dent, with paint peeling off, you'd check with friends and acquaintances to find a reliable and trustworthy auto body shop to fix it. Ignoring the problem isn't an option because it won't go away. It will only get worse, eating away at your car as rust spreads.

Yet ignoring the problem is precisely the way far too many men react when it's their bodies that are showing some rust. And that's crazy. With cash or credit, you can always buy a new car. But when *your* body goes, there's no trade-in. Heck, you can't even lease a new one.

So if you trust your favorite mechanic more than your doctor—or, worse, if you don't even have a doctor—you need to make a change. Now.

The main reason that we wrote *Symptom Solver*—and the reason that you probably bought it—is to help you help yourself. To learn to recognize what it is that your body's trying to tell you and then take appropriate action to fix the problem.

After all, that's what men do.

Neil Wertheimer
Senior Managing Editor, *Men's Health* Books

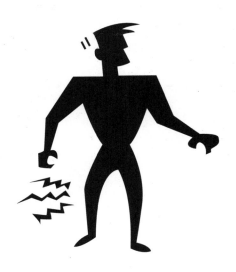

Part One

Body Talk

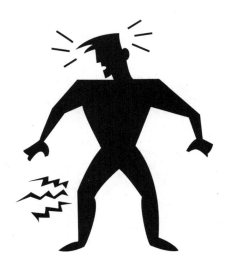

Listen to Your Body

Learn to Read the Signs

Somewhere deep within the recesses of your body is a neglected, ignored voice.

It's the voice of a doctor. And it talks to you all the time, diagnosing ailments, recommending treatments and sometimes making referrals. For instance, remember last month when you noticed that gnawing pain in your right rear molar? It kept getting worse. And the voice said, "Hey, this tooth is falling apart."

You ignored it. Hoping it would go away.

And remember when you decided it was time to get serious in the gym, and jacked up the weights while upping your workouts to five days a week? After the first three days, you had sharp pains and incredible stiffness in your arms and chest. And the voice said: "Hey, Jack. Better take a day or two off."

You ignored it. Hoping it would go away.

"We have to learn to listen to that internal doctor," says Bruce K. Lowell, M.D., an internist and geriatrician in Queens, New York, and author of *Body Signals: When to Relax, When to Be Concerned and When to Go to the Doctor Immediately.* "Men, as a rule, almost always underreact. They'll have a chest pain on a Sunday morning after not doing any activity, and they'll try to ignore it and think it'll disappear. They know inside that something is wrong. They are just afraid."

Trust Yourself

Your internal doctor uses the language of symptoms to talk with you when something's wrong. A runny nose. An achy elbow. A jackhammer headache. At times, the message is pretty clear, like the burn you feel on your skin after staying out in the sun too long. That's your inner voice's way of telling you to stay in the shade for a while. But other times, the transmission from your body may be scrambled. Dizziness, for example, can be somewhat cryptic. It could mean you're having a stroke. Or it could mean you didn't eat enough for lunch.

Think of symptoms as clues to a mystery and yourself as the bumbling Columbo trying to put together the puzzle pieces before the bad guy strikes again. The only difference is Columbo uses clues to solve murder cases and you use symptoms to solve health problems. He's just some made-up guy on TV. You're a symptom solver.

You can learn to better read the messages your body sends by following these steps.

Educate yourself. You're already ahead of the game on this one because you're reading this book. The more you learn about health, the better you'll understand your body, says Richard Honaker, M.D., of Carrollton, Texas, where he is president of Family Medicine Associates of Texas.

Pay attention. You could be a med school grad, able to identify what every textbook symptom means. But if you don't listen to your own body, all that knowledge won't do you a bit of good. The more you stop and listen to your internal doctor, the more you'll realize that you know exactly what's wrong with your body and how to fix it, Dr. Lowell says.

When in doubt, trust the voice. There may be times when your rational side is saying, "It's just a sore throat. That's no big deal." But your internal voice is saying, "I don't have a good feeling about this. There's something wrong here." This will happen more and more often as you age, primarily because the same symptom you had at age 24 does not mean the same thing when you're 54. For instance, stomach pain can have myriad causes. When you're 22, it probably means you have a virus. But at 50, it could mean you have cancer, says Dr. Lowell.

Take inventory. The best time to do this is when taking a shower. Reflect. Check yourself out. How do you feel? How do you look? "In order to be observant, people need to be intentional about it," says Robert Abel, Jr., M.D., clinical professor of ophthalmology at Thomas Jefferson University in Philadelphia, where he is one of the founders of the Alternative Medicine Program and part of a group examining the future of health care.

"You can't say, 'If it's important, then I'll see it.' You can take the same road to work every day. And one day out of a hundred you are stopped at a traffic light and you notice that there's a place that you have never seen before," Dr. Abel says. It's the same way with your body. If you drive it around in an autopilot daze, you're almost certain to miss an important road sign.

Become a body reporter. Even Jimmy Olsen, cub reporter, knows to ask the five Ws and one H: who, what, where, when, why and how. You can do the same thing with your body, says Dr. Lowell. Ask yourself questions about symptoms. The "who" should be pretty obvious. After all, it's your body. But the other questions certainly apply when a symptom occurs. How long have I had it? When does it happen? What provokes it? Where is it? The questions will do more than just bring you

You Make the Call

We thought we'd make it easy for you. We're giving you three situations. Each entails a message from your body. Here's how to interpret the messages.

1. *Situation:* Monday you were rushing off to work, ran out the front door, walked to the car and that sinking feeling hit. You just locked the keys in the house. The same thing happened Wednesday. And then on Friday, you locked them in the car. Today, you simply can't find them. Are you losing your mind?

Interpretation: You can rest easy. You probably are not senile or suffering an early onset of Alzheimer's disease. You are under a lot of stress. And that tends to reduce your present memory capabilities, says Dr. Bruce K. Lowell, an internist and geriatrician.

2. *Situation:* Last night, you and a bunch of buddies got together at the local bowling alley. This was the first time you've bowled since you were in your twenties, when—you're not shy to say—you were pretty darn good. When you awake, your chest feels tight.

Interpretation: "It's obvious that this is from bowling. You're not used to the bending down. You're not used to the heavy bowling ball," says Dr. Lowell.

3. *Situation:* You wake up on a Sunday morning. You have chest pain. You did not do any physical activity the day before. The pain persists into Monday morning.

Interpretation: If you don't get to the doctor soon, you might as well start picking out your casket. "Those are the people you hear about every once in a while suddenly dropping dead. The guy is having chest pain for six months. He doesn't tell his wife. He doesn't tell his kids. Then all of the sudden he's gone," says Dr. Lowell.

in better touch with your body; they'll also help you describe your symptoms if the pain entails seeing a doctor. "Patients don't have to be physicians. But nothing is worse than when a patient comes in and says, 'Gee, I feel lousy all over.' It means nothing. Physicians are not veterinarians," says Dr. Lowell.

When Germs Invade

Man Your Battle Stations

Germs are everywhere. On the doorknob. On the computer keyboard. On the cream cheese. On your nose.

Everywhere.

The thought is enough to turn even the most reasonable person into a neurotic, germ phobic like the wacky character that Bill Murray played in the movie *What About Bob*. He never touched anything without first wiping it off with a tissue. We'll admit, when we were researching this chapter, we were tempted to bleach everything we owned. Scrub our skin. Wear ski masks. Use tissues to turn doorknobs.

Then we talked to Ronald R. Watson, Ph.D., research professor and nutrition and immunology specialist at the University of Arizona School of Medicine in Tucson.

"Most viruses won't grow in people," he says. "They are designed to grow in plants or fungi or dogs or something else. It's only occasionally that a virus like HIV that probably was growing in a monkey or some other animal happens to mutate so that it's able to grow in a person. . . . Most of the bacteria and viruses don't bother us."

In fact, less than 1 percent of the total number of germs in the world can actually make you sick.

Whew. So all of that microscopic bacteria crawling around on our upper lips probably won't harm us. Still, 1 percent is 1 percent. And some germs in that 1 percent are pretty tough to reckon with.

You wouldn't disband an army just because most of the other countries are harmless. You'd continue to be vigilant and prepared. It's the same with your body's battle against germs. That's why we're going to let you in on a few of the germ world's best-kept secrets. Because you cannot defeat your enemy until you understand it, we'll do some basic germ reconnaissance and debriefing. Then we'll teach you some evasive tactics as well as show you how to prepare for germ warfare.

Meet the Enemy

Outside invaders lurk behind many of the most common symptoms that tell us that something has gone wrong with our bodies. From stomachaches to runny noses to fevers, scratch the surface and odds are that you'll find something that doesn't belong there. Often, the culprit is what we commonly think of as germs—bacteria and viruses. Other times, it's fungi—parasitic, spore-spewing organisms that certainly will never be confused with a "fun guy." And then there are larger parasitic creatures—ticks, worms and lice.

In scientific terms these invaders are called antigens. They trigger your immune system's automatic response alert. Let's take a closer look at them.

• *Bacteria.* These germs have it made. All they do is eat and multiply (okay, no brother-in-law jokes). Though they are too small to be seen with the naked eye, bacteria are pretty rotund germs, comparatively speaking. Thousands of viruses could fit inside one bacterium.

Inside your body, bacteria can release toxins that hinder bodily functions. They can paralyze nerves, prevent your intestines from absorbing water and generally cause havoc. But like Dr. Watson says, not all bacteria are bad. For instance, our bowels are stuffed with bacteria from our food. And the tiny creatures there help the body make vitamins, break down proteins and digest food.

• *Viruses.* They are petite, manipulative and needy. They are so small that they can't be seen under a normal microscope. They are what's known as near-life forms because they cannot fully survive on their own. Like creatures in a sci-fi flick, they need our bodies or another host to reproduce. They are made with genetic material that's similar to the genetic material in our cells. They seek out weak cells, attach themselves and then burrow into the cells' nuclei. Once there, the virus pours its DNA into the cell, instructing it to divide, thus creating more virus. The process can kill the host cell. When that happens, the original virus invades a new one.

Viruses are often responsible for respiratory tract illnesses: the common cold, sore throat and flu. When not inside a human, plant or animal body, viruses are dormant. They hang out on kitchen counters, bookshelves and other places. They are alive. But they are not reproducing.

• *Fungi.* There are thousands of these spore-producing organisms that can grow anywhere—from a slice of bread to the side of a moist shower curtain. Fortunately, most are harmless to humans. They are responsible for minor infections such as athlete's foot. Seldom do they cause deep infections except in people with depressed immune systems.

• *Parasites.* A long time ago, back when *Saturday Night Live* was actually funny (we know, some of you are far too young to remember), the late John Belushi did a skit about a guest who wouldn't leave. A parasite is like that. It uses something

Fighting Back

Pus. Fever. Swelling. They are all perils for the common, everyday germ.

If germs could think, they would see their lives flash before their cell walls when they realized the body temperature was beginning to rise, tissues were beginning to swell and some gooky yellow gunk was about to form. Pus, fever and swelling are just a few things that signal destruction for the common, everyday germ.

Take pus. It's the debris left behind after your body has battled and triumphed over some invading germs.

And fever. It means unnecessary bodily functions are slowing down so the immune system can kick into high gear. It means your bone marrow is sending out tons of cells to kill germs. It means things are heating up, an environment that simply makes life difficult for some germs.

And swelling. It means your blood vessels are leaking germ-fighting antibodies into the germ-infested area.

Are they bad reactions? "No, they're not. That all has a purpose—the pain and everything," says Terry M. Phillips, Ph.D., D.Sc., Director of Immunochemistry Labs and professor of medicine at George Washington University Medical Center in Washington, D.C.

Being laid up with a fever is about as much fun as watching a 48-hour Jerry Lewis telethon retrospective, interrupted only by commercials for psychic hot lines. But without such a defense, the various germs of the world would have killed you a long time ago.

else for its survival. And it doesn't give back anything useful in return. A virus technically could be considered a parasite by that definition. But when we're talking about parasites, we're talking about complicated organisms that are much larger than viruses: ticks, worms and lice.

Gaining Entry

From a germ's perspective, our bodies look like a well-guarded fortress. To get in, invaders first must scale a huge wall—the skin—on their way to patrolled gates—the eyes, nose, mouth, ears, anus and urethra. And the skin isn't easy to scale. It secretes sweat, which repels germ invaders even more effectively than it does other people. And body hair whisks away other invaders.

Sometimes germs get lucky. You cut yourself while chopping chicken. The bacteria on the raw meat say to themselves, "Hot dang," and make a run for the open wound. But most of the time, germs must find a way to navigate to one of the well-guarded points of entry. For them it's a waiting game. A germ may hop from the toilet paper dispenser onto a fingertip and then start pacing, tapping his foot and muttering: "I know he wants to rub his eye."

If germs are agile enough to get to our eyes, mouth, nose and other gateways, then they have more obstacles to confront. There are hairs and mucus in our passageways that can trap germs, which are then subjected to the dreaded wind torture mill. The body takes a heaving shudder and makes an intimidating "achoo" noise as a hurricane of wind rips the germ out of the mouth or nose and propels it into the air. Fluids such as saliva, sweat, tears and stomach acid can kill germs as well.

Sometimes germs get past the best guarded of nostrils, throats and other passages. And that's when the real battle begins.

The Dreaded Guinea Worm

At first read, it seems like a monster that could only spring from Hunter S. Thompson's fevered brain.

In his book *Better Than Sex*, the founding father of gonzo journalism compares politics to the guinea worm, which enters your body through drinking water and then grows inside you to more than three feet in length, "until finally it gets so big and strong that it bursts straight through the skin, a horrible red worm with a head like a tiny cobra, snapping around in the air as it struggles to breathe."

As if he already knew what we were thinking, Thompson adds, "This is true."

Considering that Thompson starts the book by recounting how he confessed to his son that he was the real gunman in the assassination of John F. Kennedy, he's not exactly the best judge to distinguish fact from fiction.

So we started sleuthing around. And we didn't have to look far. A quick computer search turned up references to guinea worms—masquerading by the name *Dracunculus medinensis*—in various medical journals. We sucked in our breath. It might really be true. We read on.

Anxiety riveted our attention. As if killer bees, great

Waging War

We're now inside the body. If a germ gets this far, it has found paradise.

"It's like going and squatting in a luxury home. You have everything, and you don't want to leave. The body is warm, comfortable and the food is in abundance," says Dr. Terry M. Phillips of George Washington University Medical Center.

So germs have developed a number of ways to go undetected. Some of them secrete a white sharks, Ebola-infested monkeys, cat-snatching pit bulls and land-encroached mountain lions weren't enough to worry about. Now we have guinea worms.

Then relief. Thompson didn't hallucinate it. It's true. But it's nothing for those of us in the Western Hemisphere to fret over. You won't have to worry about a vicious guinea worm popping out of your leg any time soon unless you plan on drinking from an infected water source in a high-risk place like India or various African countries.

In such countries the war is on to eradicate guinea worm disease. The problem is that you can drink the worm larvae. Then a year goes by. The worm grows—to more than three feet long. Then the pregnant worm realizes that its delivery date is near, so it bores its way toward the skin's surface, where it releases millions of larvae. Miraculously, less than 1 percent of the victims suffer permanent disability.

Still, it's pretty painful to have a worm use your body as a burrowing ground. Luckily, the infection can be prevented by boiling water or filtering it through a cloth. So far, Pakistan has used such methods to eliminate guinea worm infection.

waste product that is more toxic than the germ itself. The waste product acts as a smoke screen, attracting germ-killing white blood cells to it and away from the germ. Other germs are masters of disguise. They can make themselves look like something that actually belongs in the body, such as a red blood cell. Others launch a pre-emptive strike, paralyzing the immune system's ability to detect them and fight back.

That's why macrophages—a type of white blood cell—have to be such good scouts. They patrol your body in search of problems. They are constantly frisking cells, checking their molecular IDs, making sure they're not really germ spies.

When they come across some beneficial bacteria, they consult a checklist to make sure that the bugs are where they are supposed to be and in the right amount. "If they find them somewhere else, they zap them. If they find too many of them, they zap them," Dr. Phillips says.

But sometimes the macrophages encounter an enemy that they can't zap all by themselves. So they capture some of it and haul the intruder back to central command in the thymus gland, where a composite sketch of the germ is made. At central command there are two generals: a gung ho marine called the helper T cell and a laid-back, conservative suppressor T cell. The two cells look over the sketch, assess the situation and call out the ground troops known as effector T cells.

"If there are too many of these invaders, if they've gotten in the bloodstream or the generals just feel the effector T cells can't hold them off, then they call in the B cells," says Dr. Phillips. The B cells create an air strike with antibodies. The Y-shaped antibodies act like molecular rockets that spear germs two at a time. After all the germs are dead, the macrophages and another cell called a polymorphonuclear leukocyte have cleanup duty. They literally eat their dead.

Seeking Immunity

You might feel relaxed and healthy as you read this chapter, but at this very moment there are thousands of such battles going on in your body. The battlefront stretches from your head to your toes. And there are tons of casualties.

"When some of these cells are actually going into battle, they only have a life span of about 30 minutes," Dr. Phillips says.

Why don't you notice all of this carnage going on? Generally, your immune system is incredibly good at keeping germs under control. Once the immune system has triumphed over a germ, it stores that battle history in its memory. It can take anywhere from one to six weeks for your body to detect a new invader and mount an attack. But if that germ dares to invade again, it only takes two to three days. The body detects and declares war well before the germ has had a chance to multiply out of control. Also, the immune system already knows exactly how to kill that germ. It simply says, "Been there, done that." Zap. The germ is history.

Doctors can help us avoid even the initial battle with vaccinations. They inject a small amount of weakened or dead virus. The B cells easily kill it and store the battle history. So whenever a large amount of a virus such as smallpox gets in your system, your cells are already prepared for battle.

Viruses can be prevented with vaccines, but they can't be cured. Bacterial infections, on the other hand, can. When you take an antibiotic, the germs mistake it for food. For the germ, eating an antibiotic is the equivalent of us eating only potato chips. The germ eats but doesn't get nourished and eventually dies of starvation.

The Battle Plan

When you were born, your immune system had no germ-fighting memory. And you got sick. A lot. As you aged, your immune system got stronger. You got sick less often.

The problem is that the immune system doesn't continue to advance forever. Sometime in your forties, it begins to decline, Dr. Phillips says. Your T cells don't respond as quickly to

the battlefield. And by age 70, your thymus gland—your immune system's intelligence agency—is only functioning at a tenth of its effectiveness at birth.

Many doctors believe that the key to longevity is a healthy immune system. And you can slow down its demise and evade germs by following this battle plan.

Don't shake on it. Here's a scenario of how germs can spread from one person to another. A germ-free you is introduced to germ-infested Sally. Sally covers her mouth and sneezes. Achoo. Germs go from her nose to her hand. You shake her hand. They get on your hand. You see her bloodshot eyes, and just looking at them makes your eyes itch a little bit. You rub your eye with your hand. The germs get in your eye.

We're not trying to mess up your chances of getting a date with Sally or anything. For all we know she may be well worth a few days of common cold misery. But it would be a really good idea if you just didn't shake her hand, at least until she washes it. Flash her that million-dollar smile instead, and tell her in your most compassionate tone how sincerely you wish she felt better. One more thing, Dr. Phillips advises: Wash your hands often.

Halt the hanky-panky. When you feel a cold coming on, don't use a handkerchief to blow your nose. Use tissues instead. And once you blow your germs all over that tissue, get rid of it (flushing it down the toilet is a good method) so that your germs won't get someone else sick, says Dr. Phillips.

Feed the troops. They say an army marches on its stomach. The same goes for your crack germ-fighting commandos. Food can boost your immune system in two ways: taste and nutrient content. Elderly people who ate flavor-enhanced food for one study boosted their levels of B and T cells. The effect was due to the food's taste and smell, says study leader Susan Schiffman, Ph.D., professor of medical psychology at Duke University Medical School in Durham, North Carolina. The researchers weren't exactly sure why the flavor made a difference. It might be because it puts eaters in a better mood, Dr. Schiffman says.

You probably already know that your immune system needs vitamins and minerals to function properly. When you eat junk food day after day, you're essentially starving your immune system. Make sure that you get the Daily Value of all essential vitamins and minerals, especially zinc, calcium, magnesium and selenium, Dr. Phillips says. A few good ways to boost your nutrient intake include eating lots of vegetables, eating whole grains and eating breakfast every day, says Dr. Phillips.

Get off the couch. If you want the tiny warriors inside your body to be in shape, then you need to be in shape, too. That means exercise. And don't worry: We're not talking basic training here. You may have heard that exercise reduces immunity. But that's only true if you're out running marathons and biking 100 miles. For the vast majority of guys who exercise, the workouts mildly boost immunity, says Dr. Watson. The optimal amount of exercise is not known, but its main benefits are in other areas, such as reduced heart attack risk.

Snooze or lose. Ever get a cold after pulling an all-nighter? Your immune system needs rest. But it doesn't need too much rest. Shoot for somewhere between six and eight hours a night. "Lower than six and you are definitely going to get into trouble because that means you are definitely tired," Dr. Phillips says. "If you are going to sleep more than eight hours, then there is something wrong. Occasionally, ten hours is fine. But for somebody who sleeps nine or ten hours every day, that's an indication that there may be some problems."

Take a deep breath. Stress weakens the immune system. But many men still believe in toughing things out. If your job, your neighbor's barking dog or your nagging mother-in-law begin to take over your life, there's a good chance that stress is wearing down your immune system, says Dr. Phillips. Instead of pacing the floor, try some of the deep cleansing breaths that relaxation classes, books and audiotapes tell you to do. Take

deep, slow breaths, says Dr. Phillips. Let your body and mind relax. It will help you concentrate more on breathing and less on plotting your mother-in-law's demise.

Don't worry, be happy. People with a happy, upbeat attitude can produce more white blood cells than people who are despondent. So learn to laugh. Laughter decreases stress-related hormones and increases the number of T cells and B cells in the body, according to the National Cancer Institute. "Just the act of laughing can be beneficial from both an emotional and physiological perspective," says Joel Goodman, Ed.D., director of The HUMOR Project in Saratoga Springs, New York. "Physically, respiration and circulation are both enhanced through the act of laughter. We oxygenate the blood, which energizes us and helps us think more clearly."

Read the writing on the wall. There's a reason why you see those signs in the bathroom: "Employees must wash their hands before returning to work." Germs from gastrointestinal infections can get on your hands when you go to the bathroom. Then they'll get on whatever else you touch. So wash them. And don't share washcloths and other things that could pick up the same germs, says Dr. Phillips.

Revitalize with vitamins. If you're older than 60, eating healthy may not be enough to keep your immune system strong. For 29 people who participated in one study, taking a multivitamin every day for a year gave them more virile immune systems than the 27 people who took a placebo for the same amount of time. "The diets of these people were relatively good," says study leader John Bogden, Ph.D., professor of preventative medicine and community health at the University of Medicine and Dentistry of New Jersey-New Jersey Medical School in Newark. "So we think that older people either have increased requirements for some vitamins and minerals, or the Recommended Dietary Allowances each day may not be adequate to support optimal immunity in the elderly."

When Your Body Overreacts

Allergies Trip False Alarm

A blip appears on the body's radar screen. Immediately, a computer readout identifies the intruder as a virus with bad intentions. Alarms sound, and your defense system kicks into high gear. The only problem is that it's not really a virus. It's just a bunch of plant microspores that have harmlessly drifted into your airspace.

Pollen, you see, poses no real threat to your body. But in some people it sets off a reaction similar to what would happen if a virus snuck up your nose. Antibodies attach themselves to the substance, signaling mast cells to release chemicals such as histamine, which make your nose run, sneeze and swell.

All sorts of harmless substances can set off all kinds of allergic reactions. Mast cells line your nose, skin, lungs, stomach and lymph nodes. So when you eat something that you're allergic to, such as peanuts, you might get a stomachache because the peanuts interact with the mast cells in the stomach. Or, once you digest the peanuts and the digested peanuts circulate through the bloodstream, they can come in contact with mast cells in the skin, which can cause hives. Or they could circulate up to the lungs, creating wheezing. Or up to the nose, creating hay-fever-like symptoms.

"It really just depends on your body's immune system and where those cells are that are sensitive to the things that you are allergic to," says Vincent

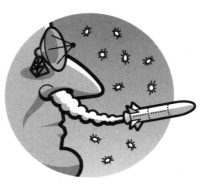

Tubiolo, M.D., a fellow of allergy and immunology at the Harbor-UCLA Medical Center in Torrance, California.

Bad Memories

Why doesn't the immune system store memory of an allergen like it does with a virus so that it can avoid the bad reaction? Well, it does. But it's not the kind of memory that you want your body to have. The first time you breathe in dust, you might not react at all. Or at least you don't notice a reaction. But your mast cells are behind the scenes at work.

They didn't like that dust. And they are plotting how to attack it in the future. So later when you breathe in dust, your mast cells respond by making your nose run and inflaming your nasal passages. "Your immune system is working against you rather than for you. It's an overreaction to things in the environment," says Dr. Tubiolo.

Doctors speculate that an allergy is a left-over defense mechanism. Some of the cells that are key in allergies are called eosinophils, which have antibodies known as IgE. The eosinophils also happen to be very good at destroying parasites.

"We think allergies were defense mechanisms first of all against parasites and also against other things that were probably harmful at one time to us, but now, as we've adapted, are no longer harmful. We no longer need protection against them. But some people still have this sensitive system that's like a hair trigger," says Dr. Terry M. Phillips of George Washington University Medical Center.

Allergy Alert

It probably won't make you feel any better knowing that you have a special antiparasite feature the next time hay fever sets in. So it's good to know that there are plenty of ways to override allergies. Here are the common ones recommended by Dr. Tubiolo.

Avoid them. Well, you could have figured that out, right? Some things you know intuitively that you're allergic to. For instance, repeated encounters with cats will be enough to let you know that their dander isn't for you. But other things aren't so easy to figure out. For instance, food. Once you eat something, it might be hours later that you break out in hives. Fortunately, food allergies are less common in adults than they are in children. But common triggers include nuts, fish and shellfish. Children are more commonly allergic to milk and soy products.

A doctor can perform a skin test that will help pinpoint your allergies. Being aware of your symptoms and what triggers them can also help doctors find the allergy culprits.

Use antihistamines. Taken orally, antihistamines can block your response to histamine. Over-the-counter antihistamines can cause drowsiness, however. Often they use the same ingredient as sleeping pills. But some antihistamines available by prescription don't cause drowsiness.

Try steroid sprays. Either inhaled through the mouth or the nose, such sprays—available by prescription—can block the response of the mast cells so that you don't get inflammation in the lungs or nose.

Have a shot. Once a doctor tests you to find out what you are allergic to, you can be subjected to a series of shots that inject increasing amounts of the allergen into your body. The idea is to inject just enough to give you a small reaction such as a hive but not

---

"Body Building"

In the beginning, there were no doctors. And it was good. If you're not convinced, read on to see what humans might look like if a bunch of British guys in white lab coats had their way.

In response to a question posed by the *British Medical Journal*, the following suggestions to "improve" the human body were made.

• No hair. Cavemen needed it to keep them warm. But now it's there just for show. Humans should be bald their entire lives.

• A head in a different place. Because they thought our heads were much too large for our poor little necks, the doctors decided to put the head within the chest, which would provide better protection for the brain. It also would make the brain more central, lessening nerve connection problems. The eyes would be on stalks connected to our shoulders, much like a garden snail's eyes. That would allow us to see in all directions.

• Better blood pumping. The doctors would replace the coronary arteries with a porous lining that would let blood move easily throughout the heart's muscle tissue. That would allow us to eat more animal fat without worrying about dying of a heart attack.

• Safer sex. To eliminate miscommunication, an area on the right shoulder would turn green when someone was thinking, "I thought you'd never ask." It would turn amber if the person was thinking, "Not now, I have a headache." And it would be red when the person was thinking, "Not if my life depended on it."

---

enough to make you feel sick. Doctors aren't in total agreement about why the shots work. But they somehow change the immune system over time. So after three to five years, a large number of patients receive significant benefits from allergy shots and may no longer need medications to control their symptoms.

When You Skip Regular Maintenance

Extend Your Body's Warranty

Whoever came up with the notion that women are "the weaker sex" must have flunked biology.

At birth, boy babies are usually thinner and biologically less mature than girl babies. More boys than girls die before their first birthday.

During adulthood, women menstruate. The monthly bloodletting makes the body constantly generate new blood. And that's healthy. Also, menstruation means that women have more of the hormones progesterone and estrogen. That keeps their good HDL cholesterol high and their bad LDL cholesterol low. And that means less heart disease, says Dr. Bruce K. Lowell, an internist and geriatrician.

So it's no wonder that women live about seven years longer, on average, than men.

Playing the Odds

In the race for longevity, men may face longer odds. That doesn't mean that they're born to lose. Men can close that gap in life expectancy with some simple body maintenance. You see, women have much more on their side than hormones. They take better care of themselves.

A few examples:
• According to one study of mortality, male death rates are higher than female death rates at every age. A prime killer of men, the study found, was something very preventable—injuries. They include suicide, car crashes, homicide and various accidents.

• Of the top ten killers of men, nine are preventable. They include heart disease, cancer, accidents, stroke, lung disease, pneumonia and influenza, AIDS, suicide and diabetes. The only cause of death officially classified as nonpreventable is homicide.

• During the past century, human life expectancy has increased by 30 years. Five of those years are the result of improved medical care, according to studies. The problem is that women have taken better advantage of such medical care than men. In 1993, women made 143 million more doctor visits than men.

"Men tend not to go to the doctor. They don't listen to their bodies. They tend not to exercise. They tend not to eat as well. There's just a whole slew of things," says Kenneth Goldberg, M.D., founder and director of the Male Health Center in Dallas and author of *How Men Can Live as Long as Women.*

By taking care of yourself, you can do more than live longer. You can live better, doctors say. And you don't have to torture yourself. It requires eating a well-balanced diet, exercising regularly, reducing stress, avoiding bad habits and seeing a doctor regularly. Yeah. We know. That sounds like a lot. But if you follow the advice in the following pages, you'll find some simple lifestyle changes that will set you on a course to a better, longer life.

Eating Right

An unhealthy diet has been linked to six of the leading causes of death: cancer, diabetes, heart disease, stroke, hardening of the arteries and cirrhosis of the liver. And obesity contributes to high blood pressure, arthritis, some cancers and heart attacks.

Fortunately, the same diet will pretty much prevent all those diseases. It's the one promoted by the American Heart Association to help prevent heart attacks: a low-fat, low-cholesterol, low-sodium diet.

Here are a few strategies to help keep your body running smoothly for years to come.

Slim slowly. In one study, men with more than a 37-inch waist were up to twice as likely to have one or more major cardiovascular risk factors as those with slimmer waists. And if your girth measures more than 39.8 inches, you're up to four times more likely to have one or more major factors for heart disease. The advice, doctors say, is simple: Lose weight.

But you don't want to take off those pounds quickly. Sudden drops in calories will send your body into starvation mode. It will reduce your metabolism and burn muscle instead of fat. So go slowly. The average man needs about 2,700 calories a day. If you eat 500 fewer calories a day than your body needs, you'll lose one pound a week, says Dr. Richard Honaker of Family Medicine Associates of Texas.

Bulk up on fiber. High-fiber diets reduce your risk of colon cancer as well as your blood cholesterol levels, says Dr. Honaker. Eat more cereals, whole-grain breads and pastas, legumes, vegetables and fruits. Other than preventing disease, the fiber will make you feel fuller faster and cut down on the time that you spend in the bathroom. Nutritionists recommend that you get at least 20 grams of fiber per day. If you start the day with oatmeal, whole-wheat toast and two pieces of fruit, you'll be halfway there.

Veg out. Eating a lot of fruits and vegetables, especially cruciferous vegetables such as cabbage and cauliflower, will reduce your risk of cancer. It also will make it easier to meet your fiber goals, says Dr. Honaker. According to the U.S. Department of Agriculture Food Guide Pyramid, you should get three to five vegetable servings and two to four fruit

servings a day. Any whole fruit, a cup of leafy greens, a half-cup of cut vegetables or fruit and three-quarters cup of fruit or vegetable juice all count as servings.

Cut fat. Fat makes you fat. It also clogs arteries, contributes to heart attacks and strokes and can thwart erections. Most men get about 40 percent of their total calories from fat. You'll want to keep your total fat intake below 30 percent of your calories, and some experts say that you should aim for 25 percent or less. On the top of the list of things to be avoided are saturated fats (those that are solid at room temperature, such as butter). Avoid fatty and cholesterol-laden foods such as eggs, red meat, fried foods, whole milk, ice cream, cheese and butter, says Dr. Honaker.

Shape Up

Before you say that you don't have enough time to exercise, think about how often you watch television. We spend about four hours a day sacked out in front of the tube. Shave just a half-hour off that and you have all the exercise time you need.

Exercise doesn't have to hurt. Just moderate activity such as walking, tennis, lawn mowing and bike riding can make a huge difference in your health, vitality and longevity, says Rex Daugherty, M.D., a physician in private practice in Pawhuska, Oklahoma. And it doesn't have to be boring. Pick an activity that you like. Then you'll be more likely to stick with it, he says.

"I tell people not to get all involved in home exercise equipment. In general, people could get more exercise if they mowed their lawns, raked their leaves, played tennis, worked on their houses and walked regularly. All of this is inexpensive. For me, exercise equipment is a drudge and usually ends up in the basement," Dr. Daugherty says.

If you are the basic couch potato type and have always had trouble sticking to an exercise routine, you might want to try breaking up the time that you exercise into short bouts. One study found that people who gradually worked their way up to four, ten-minute exercise sessions a day ended up exercising more days of the week and for a longer total time than those who exercised once a day. They also were more likely to stick with the regimen and had an easier time losing weight.

As you probably know, there are two forms of exercise: aerobic, such as running or bicycling, and anaerobic, such as weight training. With aerobic exercise, you breathe hard and your heart pounds, training your heart to pump blood more efficiently. Weight training builds muscle, which helps your body operate more efficiently and keeps you strong. Trying to decide which is best for you is like having to choose between Kathy Ireland and Elle MacPherson. Either one would be great, but having both is even better. You need 20 to 45 total minutes of aerobics and enough resistance training to target major muscle groups: back, legs, chest, arms, shoulders and abs. You'll need to do that three to five times a week, says Dr. Daugherty.

Be a Quitter

Want to live 15 minutes longer? Don't smoke that next cigarette, says Dr. Don R. Powell of the American Institute for Preventive Medicine and developer of the organization's Smokeless Program. Each cigarette takes 15 minutes off a person's life. Cigarette smoking is the leading preventable cause of illness and premature death. Smokers are 15 times more likely to get lung cancer, 16 times more likely to get bronchitis and twice as likely to have a heart attack than nonsmokers.

How to quit? Here's some advice from experts at the Centers for Disease Control and Prevention (CDC) Office on Smoking and Health in Atlanta.

Go cold turkey. Usually, if you try to stop by slowly cutting back, you'll eventually end up smoking just as much as you used to. It's the same thing with low-tar and low-nicotine cigarettes. The nicotine is so addictive that smokers who switch to lower-nicotine brands end up puffing on each cigarette harder, longer and more often.

Write it down. Figure out why you want to quit. Maybe it's to set a good example for your kids. Maybe it's to protect your family from second-hand smoke. Maybe it's to improve

Lighten Your Load

Up to 90 percent of all doctor visits are stress-related. Stress can play a role in everything from heart disease to impotence to cancer to the common cold. Some symptoms of stress include nervous ticks, throat clearing, hand clenching, feeling lonely, gritting teeth, queasy stomach, vomiting, headache, backache, neck ache, sexual difficulties, sweating, rapid heartbeat, forgetfulness, frequent urination and nightmares, says Don R. Powell, Ph.D.,

president of the American Institute for Preventive Medicine in Farmington Hills, Michigan, and author of *Self-Care: Your Family Guide to Symptoms and How to Treat Them.*

You can't eliminate stress. But you can reduce it. Here are some ideas to help you get started.

Get a hobby. But don't let it be an extension of work. If you are a chemist or accountant, try painting or bird-watching (just don't count the birds or try to figure out the probability of a bluebird sighting).

Try the 20 percent solution. Allow

your health. Now write it down and put it somewhere where you can see it. Motivation is the main component in quitting success. That's why heart attack survivors usually successfully quit. They are truly motivated. Don't wait that long.

Give it a month. You are going to have withdrawal symptoms. Some resources will help ease them, such as nicotine gum and patches. But they won't make quitting a breeze. Give yourself a month to overcome withdrawal symptoms.

Reward yourself. Celebrate each week and month that you remain cigarette-free. Count the money that you've saved by not smoking and treat yourself to something you love—other than a cigarette, of course.

Get support. There's no shortage of organizations that can help you quit. Here are some phone numbers you can call for information.

- American Cancer Society, 1-800-227-2345
- American Heart Association, 1-800-242-8721
- American Lung Association, 1-800-586-4872
- CDC Office on Smoking and Health, 1-800-232-1311
- National Cancer Institute, 1-800-422-6237

20 percent longer than originally anticipated to complete any given task. That way, you're more likely to complete your tasks on time and unstressed, experts say.

Balance your checkbook. Live within your means. A researcher at the University of Alabama studied British census data on 8,000 households and found that families that tried to maintain a lifestyle they couldn't afford were more likely to have health problems.

Get centered. One review of more than 60 studies of stress-busting tactics found that having a sense of purpose in life was the single most powerful way for men to gain peace of mind. It may come from religious involvement, from volunteer work or from political involvement. Or it may come from just sitting alone for a few minutes a day trying to work out the ways of the world—that is, to understand the cosmic significance of life and why things happen the way they do.

Avoiding the Big C

There are few words in the English language as chilling as "cancer." Only heart disease claims the lives of more men each year. So you have a choice: You can roll the dice and live in fear that cancer will one day come for you. Or you can make simple changes in the way that you live that will greatly increase the odds in your favor.

Don't fall for the line that it really is just a crapshoot. Sure, you've probably heard of some guy who smoked three packs of cigarettes a day and lived to be 100. And chances are that you've heard of another guy who did everything right and died of leukemia at age 29.

Nobody ever said that life is fair, and there are no guarantees. In some respects, whether we get cancer comes down to our genetic stock. Some people simply inherit genes that make them more cancer-prone than other people.

Still, you don't need to bank on genetics alone. There are a number of things that you can do to dramatically lessen your odds of getting cancer. But first, you need to understand what cancer is and how it works.

Cancer starts out as a copying mistake. Remember playing post office as a kid? You'd form a line and take turns whispering a message to the kid next to you. By the time it reached the end, it bore little resemblance to the original message.

That's kind of how cancer starts out. Throughout your life, your cells must make countless copies of themselves by dividing into two. And although they are pretty good at it, one in every million or so copies is different from the rest. The DNA is mutated. And that cell has a higher risk of becoming cancerous.

For that to happen, other things must go awry. Something promotes the growth of that defective cell. The promoter can come from lifestyle choices that you make, such as drinking too much alcohol or eating too much fat. Then, various cancer-fighting mechanisms built into your body must fail. That means that your immune system doesn't kill off the defective cells, and natural bodily functions that usually repair mutations somehow don't work. To put it simply, proteins that stop mutated cells from dividing are sleeping on the job.

Once cancer is allowed to grow, the mutated cells reproduce rapidly. "It squeezes out the normal cells in vital organs so that your body cannot function properly. It really invades the normal tissues and destroys the normal cells so that the body function ultimately fails," says Sidney J. Winawer, M.D., chief of gastroenterology and nutrition at Memorial Sloan-Kettering Cancer Center in New York City and co-author of *Cancer Free*.

Doctors don't have all the answers about cancer. But they do know that we are partially in control of our fates. Some of the array of malfunctions that take place to allow cancer to grow are influenced by lifestyle. For instance, doctors know that factors such as high-fat diets, smoking and alcohol consumption can make your body a more hospitable environment for cancer, says Dr. Winawer. And there probably

On the Road

Car accidents claim the lives of more men than any other type of accidental death. By now, you know to wear your seat belt, get a car with air bags, avoid drinking and driving and wear a helmet if you're on a motorcycle.

If that's all you do—prepare for that inevitable accident—you're taking a defeatist's attitude to deal with the problem. Here are some driving tips that can help you steer clear of trouble so that you don't crash in the first place, courtesy of Rick Roso, a race-car driver and spokesman for Skip Barber Driving School in Lakeville, Connecticut.

Look ahead. As you drive, look far enough into the distance so that you can see 12 seconds ahead of your car. To get an idea, pick a spot in front of you and slowly count to 12. If you reach the spot before you finish, you're not looking far enough into the distance. This will give you more time to react to problems ahead of you.

Scan. You need to take in more than just the road in front of you. Let your eyes roam from side mirror to rearview mirror to windshield so that you are aware of your surroundings. "Your eyes should never stay in one place," Roso says.

are plenty of other factors that have yet to be isolated, he says.

What you want to do is make your body a cancer-free zone. Dr. Winawer recommends the following steps to achieve that goal.

- Keep dietary fat to 20 percent of your daily calories.
- Increase your dietary fiber to 25 grams per day.
- Eat five to eight servings of fruits and vegetables a day.
- Cut back on animal products.
- Don't smoke.

Study your route. Next time you drive to work, pay close attention to the environment that you are driving in each day, from the obvious to the subtle factors that can affect your driving. That means not turning on the radio, not drinking a cup of coffee, not thinking about your job. Take in as much as you can about the route. Notice where blind intersections are located. Pay attention to where kids tend to play near the road. Look for any and all things that could possibly create a driving hazard, and make a mental note of them. You don't need to drive like this all the time. But the exercise will help you to intuitively look for trouble spots.

Drive on eggshells. When driving in slick conditions, imagine that eggs are taped to the gas and brake pedals. You don't want to break the eggs. So that means no stomping. "You breathe onto the brakes and you breathe off them. You breathe onto the gas pedal and you breathe off it. We've all gotten in cars as passengers where your head is going back and forth. The drivers don't really have a grasp of vehicle dynamics," says Roso. If you practice smoothness during dry conditions, it will be easier for you later in wet or snowy weather to maintain control of the car.

- Men are more than twice as likely to die in a motor-vehicle accident as women.
- Though more men know how to swim than women, men are nearly four times more likely to drown.
- Of all firearm-related deaths, men make up 88 percent of the victims. They are killed by bullets seven times more often than women.
- Men ages 25 to 44 are a particularly accident-prone group. Compared to women, they comprise 77 percent of the accidental deaths for that age group.

Here are a few basic safety precautions that Dr. Goldberg says can greatly increase your odds of living to a ripe old age.

- Wear your seat belt. That goes for the backseat, too. Safety belts reduce fatal injury by 45 percent.
- Don't drink and drive. About 44 percent of all traffic fatalities in 1993 were alcohol-related.
- Get air bags in your next car. Used alone, air bags are 42 percent effective in reducing moderate to critical injuries. Used with seat belts, they are 68 percent effective.
- Wear a helmet if you ride a motorcycle. Motorcycle-related deaths dropped 38 percent in California in 1992 when the state enacted a helmet law.
- Get a smoke detector and make sure it works. Homes with smoke detectors have death rates 40 percent lower than homes without them.
- If you have guns in your house, make sure everyone in the house knows how to safely handle them.

- Limit alcohol consumption to four drinks (6 ounces of wine, 12 ounces of beer or 1 ounce of spirits) a week.
- Practice safe sex. Sexually transmitted diseases can increase your risk of cancer.
- Exercise for a half-hour five days a week.
- Wear sunscreen when you're outside.

Stay Out of Harm's Way

Men are accident-prone. If you don't believe us, then consider a few statistics from the National Safety Council.

Choosing Your Doctor

How to Conduct a Thorough Examination

On the surface, doctors all look the same. They wear white coats and stethoscopes. They have horrendous handwriting. They have motel-room art, year-old magazines you wouldn't have wanted to read when they were new and syrupy elevator music in the reception area. They have a gatekeeper who wants to see your insurance card before you get your coat off. And they all have various impressive-looking framed documents and diplomas hanging on the walls.

So how do you tell one from another? And does it *really* make a difference who your doctor is?

You bet your life.

It's one of the most important decisions you can make. It's also a decision a lot of guys put off until injury or illness forces their hand. Sure, the National Center for Health Statistics in Washington, D.C., says the average man makes about 2.3 visits to the doctor per year. But that's an average: For every guy who makes four or five trips, there's one who doesn't go at all.

"A man can get to 35 years old and never see a doctor. They sometimes go longer. I see men sometimes who are in their fifties, and they tell me that they've never been to a doctor," says Dr. Bruce K. Lowell, an internist and geriatrician. "They have a million rationalizations. 'I have to work. I can't afford to take the time off.' But the bottom line is fear and denial."

A Different Kind of Checkup

As we all know, the worst time to go looking for a trustworthy car mechanic is when something's wrong with your car. So why would you wait until something's wrong with your body to find a doctor?

Take the time now to make your choice. Establishing a professional relationship and rapport with a physician can help you live a longer and more satisfying life, says Dr. Lowell. If you're confused about what to look for, read on. Despite appearances, all doctors aren't the same. Here are some key areas to examine as you make your choice.

Get on board. About two-thirds of U.S. doctors are board-certified. That means the doctor received extra training in a specialty after medical school and then passed a national exam.

"Your odds are better with a board-certified doctor. It's an important thing to look at," says Timothy B. McCall, M.D., a practicing internist in Boston and author of *Examining Your Doctor.* Some doctors claim to be certified in a specialty when, in fact, they are not, he says. You can call their bluff by checking their credentials. Call the American Board of Medical Specialists at 1-800-776-2378 to confirm board certification.

Consider a female physician. You might initially feel skittish the first time you drop your trousers in front of an adult female wearing white. But choosing a woman doctor is something to consider, says M. Robin DiMatteo, Ph.D., professor and chairwoman of the psychology department at the University of California in Riverside.

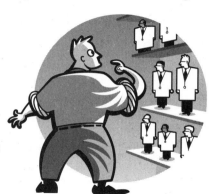

In various studies women doctors outranked their male counterparts when it came to communication skills. Women doctors also focused more on prevention. They dealt more with psychosocial aspects of health, such as family and work life. They spent more time with their patients. And they even smiled and nodded more often.

"I know several men who, after many years of going to male doctors, eventually switched to women and were a lot more comfortable. They said that the relationship was so supportive and the communication was so good that they didn't feel the least bit embarrassed," Dr. DiMatteo says.

Think young. Admit it. When you think doctor, the first image that comes to mind is Marcus Welby, M.D. Kindly. Wise. And, well, old. Possibly because new medical school courses are teaching doctors communication skills, younger doctors, on average, tend to be able to relate to patients better, Dr. DiMatteo says. They also tend to include patients more in their health care decisions rather than take an authoritarian role, she adds.

Make it convenient. If you can only go see the doctor during your lunch break and his office is closed at lunch, chances are that you'll never see the doctor. You want visits to the doctor to be convenient.

Find out the doctor's office hours, office location, billing procedures, whether testing is done at the office or somewhere else, how long you must wait for an appointment and anything else that would make seeing the doctor more convenient, says Dr. Kenneth Goldberg of the Male Health Center.

Tune in to general hospital. Hospital quality varies tremendously, Dr. McCall says. For example, the mortality rates in large teaching hospitals tend to be much lower than in small, rural, nonteaching hospitals.

Also, some hospitals specialize in treating certain conditions, and they tend to have lower mortality rates for those diseases. For instance, hospitals that do a lot of bypass

Open Wide

Wanna find a good dentist? Ask a buddy.

"The best form of referral is patient referral. You like the way a girlfriend's, father's, brother's or friend's mouth looks. They tell you that the dentist they go to is reasonable. That it doesn't hurt. You have a dentist," says Charles H. Perle, D.M.D., of the Academy of General Dentistry and the American Dental Association and a dentist in Jersey City, New Jersey.

So ask around. Get three or four names. Then call the office and ask for the office manager. Ask if the dentist has a few minutes to speak with you. Then ask him questions that are important to you. For instance, if you are afraid of needles, ask whether he can numb you some other way, suggests Dr. Perle. If you are nervous about germs and disease, ask him about his sterilization techniques.

Then on your first visit, check out the place. Make sure it's clean and presentable. Make sure you feel comfortable with the dentist.

Then go once every six months.

If you haven't been to the dentist in years, you might want to figure out why. It sounds childish, but you might be afraid. It's nothing to be embarrassed about. Dr. Perle has firefighters who would rather walk into burning buildings than sit in the dentist's chair.

If you are afraid, tell the dentist about it. He might be able to alleviate your fear. For instance, if you hate the sound of loud drills, you can ask him for a headset, says Dr. Perle.

surgery tend to have lower death rates for that surgery, Dr. McCall says.

"Part of assessing if this is the doctor for you is assessing whether this is the hospital you want to be in," Dr. McCall says. "People look at choosing a doctor, at choosing a health plan and at choosing a hospital as if they are always going to be healthy. You ought to look at doing these things as if you're going to be sick and as if you're really going to have to deal with this person."

You should make sure that the hospital where your doctor will send you is close to home, has a good reputation and has facilities to treat your specific health needs. You can call the Center for the Study of Services in Washington, D.C., at (202) 347-7283 to order a $12 book, *Consumer's Guide to Hospitals*, which contains death rates and other information about 5,500 U.S. hospitals.

Call for backup. Find out who are the other M.D.'s in the practice. Make sure you wouldn't mind being treated by them when your primary doctor is unavailable, Dr. Goldberg advises.

Check classroom attendance. You'd think no doctor would ever want to have anything to do with a classroom setting again after all those years of medical school. But doctors who want to keep up with medical advances will take a few continuing medical education courses a year. Ask any prospective doctor whether he or she takes such courses. If the answer is yes, find out which courses, Dr. Goldberg says.

Interviewing Techniques

It's role-playing time. You're a manager with the power to hire a highly skilled specialist for a position that is absolutely vital to the company's growth. After identifying the leading job candidate by

Saving Time and Money

We know that you absolutely hate waiting in the reception area. So do we. We know that you want the best medicine for your money. So do we. We know that you want to spend as little time as possible in the doctor's office. So do we.

That's why we looked into ways to make doctor's visits cheaper and more convenient. Here's what we found.

Cut the wait. Doctors can get backed up. So call ahead and ask the receptionist how the doctor is doing. "If he's 20 minutes or so off schedule, bring some work with you, or check in and run an errand in the meantime," suggests Dr. Kenneth Goldberg of the Male Health Center. By calling ahead, you've also sent the staff a subtle, but important, message: Your time is valuable, too. And they'll probably try to work you in faster.

Avoid the lunch crunch. You may save time by scheduling your appointments right after lunch. The doctor should be able to get caught up during the lunch hour. If you're the first patient after lunch, you're likely to spend less time in the waiting room.

Cut your hospital stay. If you need to schedule elective surgery, do it on a Tuesday or Wednesday. Elective surgery tends to get bumped more on Monday than any other day because of scheduling spillovers and emergency cases from the weekend. Also, you don't want your first few days of postoperative care to fall on a weekend when hospital services are reduced. Often tests and therapies that are easy to get during the week are unavailable or rare on weekends. Another consideration: Your regular doctor

reviewing credentials, what do you do?

Set up an interview. Face-to-face. And that's exactly what you need to do when you probably won't be on duty over the weekend, says Dr. Timothy B. McCall of Boston.

Get the right tests. If you have managed-care health insurance, your doctor is probably financially encouraged to order as few tests as possible. And if you have third-party insurance, your doctor is financially better off if he orders as many tests and procedures as possible, Dr. McCall says.

How do you know when you need a test? There are two ways to find out. One is to grill the doctor. Ask why he's doing what he's doing. Ask whether further testing might be necessary.

The second is to arm yourself with knowledge, Dr. McCall says. And in these times, that's a somewhat easy task. "One of the real encouraging trends right now is that consumers have access to more medical information than anytime in history with things like the Internet, consumer groups, newsletters, toll-free numbers and books and magazines," Dr. McCall says.

Pay less. Haggle. That's right. Doctor's fees are often negotiable. "It's obvious to the doctor you're a customer, so you should view him as a provider in a business relationship," says Charles Inlander, president of the People's Medical Society and author of *The Consumer's Medical Desk Reference*. For instance, if you go in with a sore throat, the doctor gives you some pills and you come back in a couple of weeks for a follow-up, don't pay the same $70 you did for the first visit. "That follow-up visit should be free of charge if the doctor finds nothing wrong," Inlander says.

free, look for another doctor. "I have had people move to town, and they have certain problems and they want to look the medical plan over. I don't think any sensible physician would charge for that," says Dr. Rex Daugherty of Pawhuska, Oklahoma.

Interviewing the doctor will help you discover something very important—his personality. And you're looking for two traits in particular.

• An ability to communicate clearly: You want your doctor to be able to explain medical terms—sigmoidoscopy, corpus spongiosum, prostaglandin—in a way that you can understand.

• A willingness to treat you like a partner, not like a child: You don't want a doctor who says, "You have pyogenic granuloma. You need surgery." You want someone who explains your condition and possible treatments and allows you to ask questions, Dr. DiMatteo says.

The doctor's ability to communicate and treat you like a partner will affect how well you respond to medical treatment, she says.

According to Dr. McCall, here are some questions you might want to ask the doctor during your interview.

• How do you feel about second opinions?
• How do you feel about non-medical treatments?
• What preventive programs would you suggest for someone my age?
• How do you feel about involving patients in decision making?

The doctor may only be able to give you five to ten minutes. So if you have easy questions that any receptionist can answer (do you take my health insurance?), then ask the receptionist.

hire a medical professional to take care of your health needs. Ask for a few free minutes of the doctor's time. If he or she won't see you for

During the interview, pay attention to whether the doctor is listening to you and whether he or she is carefully considering the questions. Look for traits that are important to you. For example, if you value a doctor who can look you in the eye when he's talking, watch his eyes.

"I think you can just get a feeling for someone. Sometimes you walk in, and the doctor and his staff are like little Napoleons and you just don't connect. Other times you feel like this is a regular person. I can deal with this person. Some of it's just a gut feeling," Dr. McCall says.

According to Dr. Don R. Powell of the American Institute for Preventive Medicine, here are some questions that you may want to ask yourself after the interview to help decide whether this is the doctor for you.

- Did the doctor listen to me and answer my questions, or was he vague?
- Do I feel comfortable with this person? Could I tell him about something personal? Could I ask something that might sound dumb?
- Is the office staff friendly?
- Could I understand what the doctor was saying?

Working Together

Okay, you're still the manager, and you've hired the employee you want based on a great interview. Now what? At most places, the person you hire comes in on probation so that you can see how he actually performs the job.

Once again, the same standard applies to your doctor.

"Ultimately, the measure of how well a doctor practices is how well a doctor practices,"

Fear and Loathing in the Reception Area

It's bad enough that everyone's taking shots at you—literally and figuratively. But if you're looking for yet another reason not to run for president, ponder this: Doctors. Lots of them.

In 1995 President Clinton was examined by an internist; an ear, nose and throat specialist; an allergist; a sports medicine specialist; a dermatologist and a nutritionist.

That's more white coats than some of us see in 30 years. Men hate going to the doctor. Just ask any man. Or any doctor. Why? Here are some theories offered by experts.

1. It's not macho. You're in your Skivvies, and he's wearing a suit. And you need this man to help you. Help is not part of the male vocabulary. If it were, we'd ask for directions every once in a while. "Many men just feel like it's a sign of weakness to complain about body illness," says Dr. Richard Honaker of Family Medicine Associates of Texas.

2. He's in control. We're not. "Most men have this feeling that they are in charge of everything. And they have trouble giving up that control," Dr. Honaker says. "In the doctor's office, they no longer run the show or call the

Dr. McCall says. "So much of the choosing we do in life, whether it's jobs or colleges or relationships, you find out what you have after you've had it for a while."

You don't, however, have to let the doctor dictate your relationship. In fact, you shouldn't. Remember, you are partially in control of how well you and your doctor get along. There are many good reasons to make sure that you establish a good relationship with your doctor. Here are a few.

- You'll more likely get special treatment. If your doctor actually knows you personally, he shots, whereas in the rest of their professional lives and in their home lives, they are telling who to do what when. All of a sudden the doctor is telling them to take deep breaths, to look to the side and cough and to get a blood test."

3. We're indestructible. Well, that's what we like to think. We like to think that we're so strong, nothing can overpower us. "There's a belief that men are invincible—bulletproof," says Dr. Kenneth Goldberg of the Male Health Center.

4. It's new territory. Unlike us, women grow up learning to deal with doctors. They need Pap smears. They need breast exams. They need the doctor to prescribe birth control. They need the doctor to deliver their babies. They need the doctor to inoculate their babies.

"I think women kind of get used to going to the doctor out of necessity. Men generally don't encounter significant problems until their middle years," says Dr. Rex Daugherty of Pawhuska, Oklahoma.

5. We want to try it our way. Dr. Daugherty offers this example about men: "If they get to where they can't urinate well and they are 50 or 60 years old, they will say to themselves, 'This will start clearing up if I just stop drinking coffee and soda.' They will try all of these things until some morning when they get up and they cannot urinate at all. Then they will go see the doctor."

will be more likely to agree to schedule changes, to make an exception to the rule or arrange for after-hour calls, Dr. Daugherty says.

• You'll listen. About 38 percent of patients don't follow short-term advice from their doctors, and 43 percent don't follow long-term advice. In various studies, Dr. DiMatteo has found that part of the problem is that the patient doesn't understand what the doctor says and is too timid to ask questions. Having a good relationship with your doctor, where you treat one another as health partners, will help alleviate your shyness, she says.

• You'll get better. Fully discussing the situation with your doctor can make the difference between getting cured and staying sick. In one study, headache sufferers whose symptoms improved the most during a six-month period were the ones who discussed their symptoms the most fully with their doctors at the first visit.

"Patients are less likely to volunteer symptoms if the doctor is trying to act like their parent," says Dr. Richard Honaker of Family Medicine Associates of Texas. "But male patients respond better if they feel like the doctor is a business partner. It would be like the doctor and patient were discussing an issue about the business. It happens to revolve around his stomach or his nose or his throat."

So start acting like your doctor is your business partner. If your accountant started throwing around technical terms and mumbo jumbo about numbers, you'd stop him and demand: "What does that mean? What's the bottom line?" Do the same thing with your doctor.

And don't be afraid to take the initiative. You may have read about a nutritional therapy that your doctor doesn't know about. Instead of waiting for him to bring it up, ask him whether eating an apple a day will keep the tennis elbow away. He might answer, "Uh, dunno." Then say that you're willing to try it. And ask whether he'd be interested in hearing about your progress, suggests Thomas Jefferson University's Dr. Robert Abel, Jr. He is also a key player in Jefferson's Alternative Medicine Program, which is examining the future of healing in the twenty-first century.

"If you are told, 'Inquire wherever you want. Whatever information you can find, I would like to hear about it'—that's the kind of doctor you want to be with," Dr. Abel says.

Getting What You Need

Here are a few ways you can make sure that you stand up for yourself.

See your doctor. The more you do it, the easier it will get, Dr. Honaker says.

Remember who pays the rent. His rent. And the answer is: You do. Remind yourself of this fact. Either you or your health insurance company is forking out a wad of cash every time you see the doctor. This isn't charity work. The doctor needs you and your money, so don't ever feel that you're wasting his time.

"Whether it is a large or small concern, the physician should listen to the patient and see what can be done. I never feel like my time is wasted by any patient," Dr. Daugherty says.

Fly solo. Women have more experience with doctors. So having your spouse in the examining room with you may increase your chances of getting the right questions asked. Then again, some wives take over the visit.

Instead of letting their husbands talk, it's the wives who describe the symptoms. And they tend to exaggerate, Dr. Lowell says.

"Wives are getting their information secondhand. And they know their husbands never complain. So they take it for granted that if the husband is complaining, the pain has to be a lot worse than he says it is," Dr. Lowell says.

It may sound like good fodder for a sitcom, but Dr. Lowell has actually watched husbands and wives heatedly argue about what type of pain the husband is feeling.

Go to rehearsal. Before you even step into the doctor's office, rehearse what you want to say, Dr. DiMatteo advises. And if it's your first visit, be prepared to talk about the following: your medical history, your dietary habits, your occupation, your sleep habits, any family problems, your lifestyle, your stress level and your attitude toward health.

Make a list. It works for Santa. It can work for you. Write down whatever it is you want to be sure to tell the doctor and bring it with you. When listing symptoms, be as specific as possible. Even write the date and time each one occurred. List what you want to talk about in descending order of importance. Sending your list to the doctor ahead of time is even more effective, says Dr. Abel.

Don't feel rushed. It seems like the doctor is always in a hurry. And that hurriedness may make you feel like he doesn't have time for your piddling little question. That's not true.

"I'm going to tell you a secret about medical practice. You know how doctors are always rushing from one room to another? And they seem to be rushing so they can go take care of really sick people or people with emergencies? They really are rushing to the next patient because the more patients they see, the better their income," Dr. DiMatteo says.

Now if Joe Towe in the next room has an ingrown toenail, then Joe's toe can wait. "You have just as much right to the doctor's time as anybody else," Dr. DiMatteo says.

Be persistent. So you tell the doc, "Hey, don't leave yet. I have an important question." He tells you he has a patient backlog that's 12 days long. And you don't want to push it. Then ask if there's someone else in the practice you can talk to—a nurse, a health educator, a dietitian. Or ask him to refer you to written information. Or a support group. Or make another appointment with the doctor, says Dr. DiMatteo.

"You have to get your questions answered. If the doctor doesn't answer your questions, you're going to end up with a lot of trouble down the road," she adds. "Often the doctors don't make those referrals because they think patients don't want them. I think just by being direct the patient gets the doctor's attention."

Follow through. If you leave the office with unanswered questions, send a follow-up letter. In it, you can summarize what the doctor said to make sure that you got it straight as well as question him further.

"Believe it or not, anyone who takes the

time to write something down gets a response," Dr. Abel says. "But a phone call is random. You may get called back at a time you are not thinking about things. You feel like you've interrupted somebody else's schedule. You are embarrassed. So you hurry. Then you forget to ask something."

Act like a parrot. Repeat what the doctor has told you to do. It will let the doctor know whether you understand, Dr. Powell says.

Speak up. So the doctor is telling you how eating a head of cauliflower every day for a month will get you back in tip-top shape. You're nodding your head, but all you can think is: "I hate cauliflower."

Tell the doctor. If you don't, he'll assume you're on that cauliflower diet when you're not. Then when you return a month later and you're still sick, he'll prescribe something stronger— perhaps a head of broccoli to go along with it. Or, worse, he'll think he misdiagnosed you and order up a battery of tests to find out your real problem.

Sweeten him up. In one study, when internists were given small bags of candy as gifts, they performed much better on tests of problem-solving ability than doctors who didn't receive anything. Even simply saying thanks when he helps your ills go away can go a long way to improving your care. "Acknowledge your doctors' accomplishments and tell them when they're doing good work," says Alice M. Isen, Ph.D., professor of psychology at Cornell University in Ithaca, New York. "Too often we only give feedback when things aren't working."

Stay calm. In one study, internists were shown a videotape of someone portraying a patient with chest pain. When the patient spoke in a controlled, businesslike manner, half the internists correctly diagnosed heart disease as the culprit.

Room Service

Getting sick or injured on a business trip used to mean a trip to the emergency room. But now, you can call HotelDocs at 1-800-468-3537, and—in about the time it takes to have a pizza delivered—a doctor will be at your hotel room.

A dispatcher will take your medical information and send a physician, dentist or specialist to your hotel room within 35 minutes. The doctors supply the medications, so you don't have to hunt for a pharmacy. The exam charge is about $150 and is covered by most insurance plans. HotelDocs' doctors are available 24 hours a day, seven days a week in 40 cities nationwide.

But when the patient described symptoms with excited emotional gestures, only 13 percent of a different group of doctors came to the same conclusion. The majority of those doctors diagnosed the patient as having an anxiety attack.

Tell him off. You don't have to be a bully about it, but if you find that your doctor repeatedly doesn't answer your questions, then tell him about it. Give the doctor a chance to change.

"Some doctors are willing to change," says Dr. DiMatteo. "Say, 'I don't like a relationship where things are one-sided. I really want to be a participant, and I think I can be a better patient and take better care of myself if you answer my questions and we can talk about different strategies and possibilities for my care.' "

If the doctor doesn't change, that means it's time to find a new one, says Dr. DiMatteo. If you find yourself in that position, go back to the beginning of this chapter and start all over again.

When to See Your Doctor

Symptoms That Scream "Get Help"

So one morning you wake up, roll out of bed and start the normal routine. You walk to the bathroom, stand in front of the toilet and take aim. Instead of a normal, forceful stream, you get an on-again, off-again trickle.

You know that you have to urinate. But it just doesn't want to come out.

Do you:

a. call your doctor?

b. wait and see if the same thing happens tomorrow?

If you're like most guys, you wait until the next day. And the next. Meanwhile, inside your body, your prostate continues to swell. You wake in the middle of the night. You go to the bathroom. You wait. It trickles. You wait. It trickles. You still don't go to the doctor. Your prostate swells some more.

You ask your sister what she thinks. She tells you to drink some cranberry juice. It doesn't help. Your prostate swells some more, blocking the urine from getting out of your bladder. One Sunday afternoon your prostate has become so large and so much urine is backed up in your bladder that you feel pain unlike any pain you've ever felt before. You call your doctor. But he's at a golf resort where there are no telephones. You go to the emergency room.

"For men, going to see the doctor is the last resort," says Dr. Rex Daugherty of Pawhuska, Oklahoma.

But it shouldn't be.

All too often men know something's wrong. And we figure we can tough it out. The problem gets worse. And by the time we drag ourselves in to see the doctor, he either can't do much for us or must resort to an undesirable method of treatment—surgery. But if we had dragged ourselves in sooner, the problem could have been alleviated.

Don't Think—Just Go

It's okay to ignore an occasional ache or pain that goes away as quickly as it comes. But when something is clearly out of the ordinary, your body is telling you to get help, says Dr. Kenneth Goldberg of the Male Health Center. "In general, when things are different in the body, there's a reason to want to explore it," Dr. Goldberg says. "We're not talking about a headache that lasts for two minutes and is gone forever. We're talking about someone who repeatedly gets a headache."

Here are some symptoms that you should *never* ignore. They all scream one thing and one thing only—go to the doctor.

• Chest pain. Seems obvious, right? But many men have heart attacks and ignore the symptoms. They think that it's heartburn, says Dr. Richard Honaker of Family Medicine Associates of Texas. "If it's a dull, squeezing pain in the mid-chest that lasts longer than a few minutes and is accompanied by shortness of breath, a cold sweat and nausea, and pain that radiates to the left arm or jaw, it's probably your heart," he says. "But there are variations on that theme. A man shouldn't even try to decide whether he should or shouldn't go to the doctor. He just should see a doctor if he has chest pain or vague chest discomfort."

• Severe shortness of breath. It's normal to get winded after climbing a flight of stairs. But if you find yourself gasping for air for no reason, call your doctor. Even without chest pain, you could be having a heart attack, says Dr. Goldberg in his book *How Men Can Live as Long as Women*. It can also be a sign of asthma or lung disease.

• Blood. If someone wallops you in the nose and it bleeds a bit, you know what's going on. Unless, of course, you're on the canvas, and a guy in a sharp bow tie is standing over you, counting loudly to ten. We're talking about seeing blood when there's no obvious reason for it to be there. Like when you cough up blood or find it in your stool or urine. "The thing that generally will bring the most stoic man to the doctor's office is the sight of blood. Still, a lot of people say, 'Gosh, I have a cold. I've been coughing real hard. I probably just popped a little blood vessel in one of the bronchial tubes.' Or when they find blood in the stool they think it's from hemorrhoids," says Dr. Daugherty. It's possible that the cause is that benign. But it's also possible that you have cancer, Dr. Daugherty says.

• Dizzy spells. We're not talking about the ones that happen after you've been lying on the couch all day and then suddenly get up to answer the phone. And we're not talking about alcohol-induced bed spins. We're also not talking about how you feel after riding the Gravitron at an amusement park.

We're talking about regular dizzy spells. "If you have it pretty much every day or every week, and you notice that your vision is a little funny or that you are nauseated, it could be an early warning sign of a stroke," says Dr. Daugherty. Often, as small blood vessels in your brain get closed off, they'll send you such warning signs months in advance. Other signs of stroke include sudden weakness or

Prescription for Saving Money

The most important thing to remember when your doctor hands you a prescription is this: Ask questions. It will save you money.

"You have to remember the incredible influence of the pharmaceutical industry over what drugs are prescribed," says Dr. Timothy B. McCall of Boston. "When a doctor prescribes an antibiotic that sells for $90 for a week's worth of pills, you know it is brand new.

"It's the highly promoted medicines that are so darn expensive. As soon as there's a generic equivalent, the price will drop to a half or a third," Dr. McCall says. "There are times when you need these drugs. But in general, new drugs end up being prescribed when older, safer drugs—which happen to be a lot cheaper—would be better."

According to Dr. McCall, to get the best drugs for your money, you should ask the following questions.

- **How new is this drug?**
- **Is there a cheaper or generic equivalent available that would work as well as this drug?**
- **What's the long-term safety of this drug?**
- **Is there a reason that this new drug has an advantage over older, safer drugs?**

numbness on one side of the face, loss of speech and sudden severe headache.

• No healing powers. If you cut yourself and it takes longer than normal to heal, it could mean that your immune system isn't working properly, says Dr. Terry M. Phillips of George Washington University Medical Center. Other signs of an impaired immune system include skin boils and random colds.

• Impotence. If you continually have trouble getting and maintaining erections, it could be an omen of other health problems.

Clogged arteries, high blood pressure and dia-betes can cause impotence. One in four men who see a doctor because they have a potency problem will have a heart attack or stroke within five years.

• Lingering illness and fever. Now, you don't need to go to the doctor every time you feel a sniffle coming on. First of all, if you have a cold or the flu, the doctor can't do much for you but tell you to rest and drink a lot of liquids. But if your coldlike symptoms last longer than three days, are accompanied by a fever higher than 101°F or rapidly intensify, then you should see your doctor, advises Dr. Honaker.

• Thirst coupled with lots of trips to the bathroom. There are four signs of diabetes: constant thirst, frequent need to urinate, fatigue and weight loss. If you have two of these symp-toms, you should see your doctor, says Dr. Goldberg.

Check It Out

Don't you just hate how your wife or girl-friend will nag you about going to get a check-up? Well, she might not be totally to blame. Her doctor just might have put her up to it.

"The way I get men to come in for their physicals is I talk to their wives," says Dr. Honaker. "I'm not being facetious. That's what works."

But your wife and your doctor do have a point. There are lots of reasons why you should see the doctor even when you don't feel the slightest bit under the weather.

"Many diseases are silent. They are only discovered by things that we do to look for them, not things that you as a man can feel," Dr. Honaker says.

For instance, about 30 percent of men over age 50 have polyps in their colons. They can't feel a thing. But the lumps are there. Some of those growths will turn into cancer. If you go in for regular checkups, your physician can find such growths through a procedure called

sigmoidoscopy. Then he can take them out painlessly before they have a chance to become cancerous, Dr. Honaker says.

For those who don't get routine checkups, "the price they pay is three to five years later, they may have colon cancer that could have been prevented," Dr. Honaker says.

Think of your body as a car. The owner's manual tells you to take your car in for regular maintenance checks after you've traveled so many thousand miles. You wouldn't skip the checks just because your car isn't making strange noises. Well, that's the same thing with your body, says Dr. Honaker. Men ages 15 to 39 should get a physical every three years. Those ages 40 to 49 should have one every two years. And those age 50 and above should go once a year.

When you go in for a physical, your doctor will conduct an array of tests. Doctors know that all that probing and exploring makes us uneasy. But with a little education and prac-tice, routine checkups become just that: routine. So here are some basic medical tests, why they are important and how often you should make sure you get one.

Rectal exam. This and this alone is probably one of the biggest reasons why you haven't been to see the doctor lately. But a lot of the aversion to the test can be eliminated with education and practice, doctors say. When the doctor inserts his lubricated, gloved finger into your rectum, he's feeling your usu-ally soft prostate. He's searching for any pea-size nodules or tumor masses that could mean cancer, says Dr. Daugherty. The doctor also will remove some stool to examine it for blood.

Relaxing by taking some deep breaths and making sure not to clench your fists or grab the table will help the doctor get the job done more easily. Also, seeing the same doctor regu-larly will reduce some of the embarrassment, Dr. Daugherty says.

"Now nobody enjoys this any more than a woman enjoys a vaginal examination. But women are more used to vaginal examinations than men are to rectal examinations. That's the reason men always speak of it with such disdain," says Dr. Daugherty.

The American Cancer Society recommends that men older than 40 should have a rectal exam once a year, says Dr. Goldberg.

Sigmoidoscopy. It's a big word. And it's probably less scary if you don't know what it means. If there's anything more dreaded than a rectal exam, it's this. The doctor uses a lighted, thin, flexible instrument called a sigmoidoscope to look inside your rectum, colon and large intestine. It's a more precise test than the rectal exam and is used to diagnose colon cancer and polyps in the earliest and treatable stages.

Men older than 50 should get one every three to five years, says Dr. Honaker.

Urine test. You know the drill: Take the plastic cup, head for the bathroom. The sample lets the doctor know how well your body gets rid of waste. Among other things, the doctor can check for diabetes, infection, cancer and kidney stones. You should have one with every physical exam, says Dr. Goldberg.

Blood test. The doctor can check for a lot of things by looking at your blood. But we're going to talk about only two here. The first is blood cholesterol. The test is called a lipid profile, and it helps the doctor find out how much of the bad LDL, plaque-forming blood cholesterol you have compared to the good HDL cholesterol, which seems to combat plaque. You want your total cholesterol to be under 200.

The second blood test looks for prostate-specific antigen (PSA), which is made by your prostate gland. Levels of the antigen rise when

What's Up, Doc?

If you can't figure out what your doctor wrote on your prescription, it may be because you don't speak the language. Doctors use their own form of shorthand, says Dr. Don R. Powell of the American Institute for Preventive Medicine in his book *Self-Care: Your Family Guide to Symptoms and How to Treat Them*. Now, you could hire a translator, but prescriptions already cost way too much. So we'll make it easy for you. Here are some translations for common abbreviations that doctors use.

ad lib.	as needed
a.c.	before meals
b.i.d.	twice a day
caps.	capsule
gtt.	drops
h.s.	at bedtime
p.c.	after meals
p.o.	by mouth
p.r.n.	as needed
q.4.h.	every four hours
q.d.	daily
q.i.d.	four times a day
q.o.d.	every other day
t.i.d.	three times a day
Ut dict., UD	as directed

there is something wrong such as infection, prostate enlargement or cancer. A normal PSA is less than 4.

You should have your PSA checked once a year starting at age 50, says Dr. Goldberg.

Testicular exam. This probably is more embarrassing than anything else. The doctor feels your testicles for lumps that are signs of cancer. This should be done during your physical exam by your doctor, and once a month you should do a testicular self-exam.

When to Get a Second Opinion

You probably thought seeing one doctor was bad enough. But there are times that you'll want a second doctor's opinion. And don't feel embarrassed about asking for one.

"A doctor ought to view a second opinion as the opportunity to learn from a colleague rather than a threat," says Dr. Timothy B. McCall of Boston.

Obviously, any time your doctor recommends that someone stick a scalpel inside your body, you should get another opinion. But, according to Dr. McCall, there are lots of other reasons to consult another doctor.

- Whenever you are facing any extreme treatment—chemotherapy, for instance
- Any time your doctor recommends a very expensive or very invasive test
- Your gut feeling is that your doctor is missing something
- You don't feel that your doctor is taking your symptoms seriously
- You think that you should be getting better, but you are not
- Whenever your doctor says you might have something but he just isn't sure— for example, if a pathologist says that your biopsy results may or may not show cancer

If you have health insurance with a health maintenance organization (HMO), you won't have as much choice in doctors. But this might be a time when you want to find a doctor outside your medical plan and pay out of your pocket, Dr. McCall says. Often, doctors in HMO plans have financial incentives to recommend the least expensive treatments—not necessarily the best. So if you think you need surgery, you

---

Take Your Best Shot

A trip to the doctor's office each fall for a flu shot may save you several trips—and a lot of misery—each winter. The flu is responsible for 10,000 to 40,000 deaths, 150,000 hospitalizations and countless missed work and school days a year. It costs consumers $12 billion annually.

Studies show that getting a flu shot reduces your sick days from work as well as your visits to the doctor—with one study finding a net annual savings estimated at $47 per vaccinated person.

---

may need to go outside the plan to find someone else who thinks so, too, Dr. McCall says.

"If you get somebody outside the plan who says, 'Listen, you need to have this done,' that gives you the ammunition to go back to your plan and say, 'This person said this. Why aren't you doing this?' It may cost you a few hundred bucks. But if there's a lot at stake, it may be worth it to you," Dr. McCall says.

What if you get two totally different recommendations? How do you know which doctor is right? Well, a lot of it is gut feeling. But there are a few things that Dr. McCall says you should keep in mind. Any doctor who works for an HMO has an incentive not to recommend surgery. So if he tells you to check into the hospital pronto, you can be pretty sure that you need to go. Then again, surgeons perform surgery for a living. If you ask a surgeon if you need surgery, chances are that he'll find something to operate on.

"Surgeons believe in surgery. That's what they do," Dr. McCall says. "Get a second opinion on surgery from a nonsurgeon. Don't go to another neurosurgeon to ask him about your back surgery. Go to a neurologist. Don't go to a second cardiac surgeon. Go to a cardiologist."

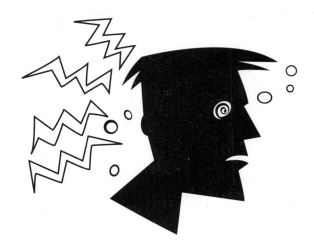

Part Two

Head

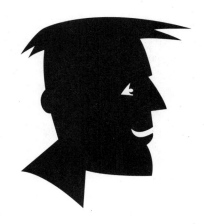

Bad Breath

• When you roll over to kiss your wife good morning, she jumps out of bed

• People always give you more than enough personal space

• You rub a cotton swab around the inside of your mouth, including your gums and tongue; when you sniff the cotton swab, you almost pass out

What It 💭 Means

If you can't tell Orel Hershiser from oral hygiene, odds are that you have bad breath. Even if you can, and you brush and floss regularly, you might not be doing it correctly, says Cherilyn G. Sheets, D.D.S., of the Academy of General Dentistry and a dentist in Newport Beach, California.

Improper brushing and flossing can allow bacteria to accumulate in your mouth like mildew on a shower curtain. If you don't get rid of the bacteria, it'll start to smell as it rots leftover food particles. This leads to gum and tooth disease, which smells even worse, says Charles H. Perle, D.M.D., of the Academy of General Dentistry and the American Dental Association and a dentist in Jersey City, New Jersey.

Bad breath also can be caused by stomach discomfort, postnasal drip and certain foods, such as garlic and onions.

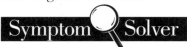

Symptom Solver

Avoiding foods that smell—garlic, onions, fish—is always a good idea. And we don't need to tell you that brushing (don't forget your cheeks and tongue) and flossing are essential. It also helps to gargle with a non-alcohol-containing mouthwash, says Dr. Sheets.

If those remedies are already part of your daily routine, but they don't work, try this.

Make yourself see red. Swish about a teaspoon of red food coloring in your mouth after brushing and then spit it out. The red spots it leaves behind will highlight the spots you missed when brushing, says Dr. Perle. Just be sure to put some petroleum jelly on your lips first or you'll turn them red, too, he cautions.

If all your best efforts come to naught, you should demonstrate your technique in front of a dentist or dental hygienist to make sure that you're doing it right, says Dr. Sheets.

Sometimes—like when you're deer hunting in a dense Pennsylvania forest and you realize you forgot your toothbrush—you have to be resourceful. And there are ways to freshen your breath without brushing. Just remember: These are merely quick fixes. They are not—repeat *not*—a substitute for regular brushing and flossing.

But if you discover that you've been afflicted with a malodorous mouth moments before an important meeting with the boss—or just as you've finally worked up the nerve to ask out that gorgeous brunette in the sales department—here are some hints to help you breathe easily.

Munch a bunch. Some foods will mask bad breath. Chewing on parsley or mint are temporary solutions, Dr. Sheets says. You also can try peppermint or anise.

Other foods can stimulate saliva production, which rinses your mouth of offending bacteria, says John D. McDowell, D.D.S., assistant professor in the Department of Diagnostic and Biologic Sciences at the University of Colorado School of Dentistry in Denver. They include crunchy vegetables and citrus fruits.

Rinse. Swish some water vigorously and then spit to wash away food and crank up your saliva production. Even simply drinking water will help to keep that smelly bacteria on the move, says Dr. Sheets.

Buy gum. Chewing sugarless gum stimulates saliva and keeps bacteria at bay, says Dr. McDowell.

Bleeding Gums

- Swollen, reddish or painful gums
- Gums that bleed easily

What It ❓ Means

Ever have someone nag you to do something for your own good? You don't necessarily want the advice, but you know, deep down, that it's worth paying attention to.

Maybe it's time that you listened to your gums. When they get red, puffy and bloody, they are nagging you to take care of your mouth. Sure, you can ignore them—if you're willing to spend the rest of your life looking like a washed-up hockey player.

Bad gums are generally caused by plaque, a sticky, invisible substance that sticks to the teeth. Over time the plaque hardens into tartar. Both plaque and tartar irritate the gums and may gradually eat away the bone to which your teeth are anchored. That's why you should listen to your gums' cries for help.

Symptom 🔍 Solver

You can reverse gum disease if you catch it early, says Dr. Charles H. Perle of the Academy of General Dentistry and the American Dental Association. Start with the advice that you've probably heard a zillion times: Brush and floss every day and have your teeth professionally cleaned twice a year. And we'll show you a few ways to take better care of your mouth, including how to make brushing and flossing easier and more effective.

Feel the burn. Food isn't always your friend. Two of the painful problems that it can cause go by the highly technical medical names popcorn-kernel syndrome and pizza burn.

When food particles like popcorn kernels get wedged beneath the gum, "the gum will circle around it and become inflamed and puffy," Dr. Perle says.

And hot foods can burn the heck out of your mouth. You might be thinking coffee, tea or soup. But the biggest offender, dentists say, is pizza. The cheese can get so hot that it chars the skin on the roof of the mouth, says Dr. Perle.

To treat popcorn-kernel syndrome, remove the particle with a toothpick or floss. Then follow the Rolling Stones' advice and let it bleed; the blood will flush the area, Dr. Perle says. For pizza burn, the best thing that you can do is let it heal on its own. Or rub on a little benzocaine oral cream, such as Orajel or Anbesol, to help ease the pain.

Do the test. How much plaque is on your teeth? After brushing, put some petroleum jelly on your lips, swish about a teaspoon of some red food coloring in your mouth, then spit it out, says Dr. Perle. (You can also ask your dentist for a disclosing tablet, which does the same thing.) The food coloring makes plaque stain red, showing you where you missed brushing, Dr. Perle says. Don't panic if you see red. If you go back and brush away the red, you've brushed away the plaque.

Work in shifts. If you've just started flossing, don't be surprised if pulling the string between your teeth causes bleeding. It takes time to floss gums into shape, so start slowly. Floss a few teeth at a time. Start with the back teeth, since they tend to be in worse shape than those in front, says Dr. Cherilyn G. Sheets of the Academy of General Dentistry.

When you can floss those teeth with little or no bleeding, move on to the next section and then the next until you're doing your whole mouth at one time, Dr. Sheets says.

Make a date. Flossing at the same time every day will make it part of your routine—like undressing before getting into bed—so that you're less apt to forget it, says Dr. Sheets.

Replace your gear. Don't wait until your toothbrush is down to three bristles before replacing it. Buy a new one every three to six months, says Dr. Perle. You may even want to replace it sooner if the bristles start to bend.

Canker Sores

- You have small white or gray sores on the inside of your mouth
- You have a tingling or burning sensation

What It Means

Doctors are not sure what causes canker sores. It could be that the immune system is temporarily weakened. Stress may play a role. It could be an amino acid imbalance. It could be an injury—caused, say, by biting your lip while eating a carrot. It could even be a diet that includes too many acidic foods.

To make an uncomfortable situation worse, canker sores often pop up two to three at a time; some people get as many as 15 or more. When you get them, there's no reason to be alarmed. They pose no serious health threat. They are basically a big pain in the mouth.

Symptom Solver

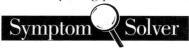

It's an old adage among dentists: You can treat a canker sore for a week, or wait for it to go away on its own in seven days, says Dr. Charles H. Perle of the Academy of General Dentistry and the American Dental Association.

Even though canker sores will go away on their own—with or without treatment—there are ways to make them go away faster, and also to relieve pain in the meantime, says Dr. Cherilyn G. Sheets of the Academy of General Dentistry.

Use a medication combo. To ease the pain of canker sores, rinse your mouth with a half-and-half mixture of Kaopectate and Benadryl liquid. Swish the concoction in your mouth for at least a minute before eating. The Benadryl will numb the pain, while the Kaopectate helps the anesthetic stick to the inside of the mouth, says Louis M. Abbey, D.M.D., professor of oral pathology at Virginia Commonwealth University/Medical College of Virginia School of Dentistry in Richmond.

Take your mouth for an ocean swim. Rinsing your mouth with some salt water several times a day will help ease the pain of canker sores, says Eric Z. Shapira, D.D.S., a dentist in private practice in Half Moon Bay, California. Mix a teaspoon of salt in an eight-ounce glass of warm water and swish it around in your mouth, he advises.

Hold the spicy foods. Acidic or spicy foods, such as orange juice, tomato sauce and grapefruit, can make a canker sore burn like fire. You don't need a doctor to tell you that; your mouth will do it for you. But there's a more important reason to forgo the fiery foods: If you have frequent canker sore outbreaks, the foods can actually set off attacks. "It hurts *and* it activates it," says Dr. Sheets. "People who have very acidic diets are more prone to breaking out in canker sores."

Try lysine. Some canker sore sufferers may have an amino acid imbalance—too much arginine and not enough lysine, says Dr. Sheets. In one small study, people who took two 500-milligram lysine tablets every six hours had their canker sores heal more quickly than those who didn't take the supplements.

Lay off. When you feel one of those whitish bumps on the tip of your tongue, there's an urge to use your front teeth to bite down on it. Don't. All that biting and gnawing will make the canker sore more inflamed, says Dr. Sheets.

Ask for help. If you get canker sores a lot, you can ask your dentist to prescribe triam-cinolone acetonide (Kenalog) in orabase, says Dr. Sheets. Two to three times a day, use a towel to dry off the lesion and then apply enough of the ointment to thinly coat the sore. Make sure to put it on after meals so that your food and drink don't wash it off. The small amount of antibiotic in the prescription will help it heal faster and eliminate secondary infection, says Dr. Sheets.

Chapped Lips

- Your lips are dry and cracked

What It ? Means

Lips are a lot like car paint. You park your car outside day after day. It rains. Your car gets wet. The wind blows. Your car gets dry. It rains. The wind blows. You look at your car, and you think one thing: "Wax."

Your lips go through much the same torment as your car paint, especially during cold weather. Lips chap because, unlike the skin on the rest of your body, they lack natural oils needed to protect them against frigid winds and low humidity.

They also are easily burned by the sun's rays because they don't have melanin, the pigment in the rest of the skin that helps to screen out sunlight.

Symptom Solver

Probably the easiest solution for your lips is the same one you use for your car: Wax them. Apply lip balm every hour or two. And make sure to use it at bedtime.

"While most people remember lip balm when they are facing the elements, they may not realize that we can lick our lips in our sleep," says Anita Cela, M.D., clinical assistant professor of dermatology at Cornell University Medical College in New York City.

The waxy ingredient in lip balms is all pretty much the same, says K. William Kitzmiller, M.D., volunteer clinical professor of dermatology at the University of Cincinnati and spokesman for the American Academy of Dermatology.

But you should look for a balm that has a sun protection factor (SPF) of 15 or higher to block out the sun's rays. And use it year-round. That will protect you against skin cancer.

"Often, once men reach age 60 or 70, they get precancerous lesions, usually on the lower lip, from years of sun exposure," says Mitchell C. Stickler, M.D., a dermatologist in private practice in the beach community of Lewes, Delaware.

Here are some other ways to pay lip service.

Keep your tongue in your mouth. Any wetting and then drying will dry out skin, says Dr. Stickler. So tell your tongue to keep off. Using a lip balm will help you restrain yourself.

Breathe through your nose. Winter air is cold and dry. When you suck it in through your mouth, you'll dry your lips, Dr. Kitzmiller says. And the air you breathe out has moisture. It will wet your lips, which is almost as bad as licking them. So try to breathe through your nose.

Switch toothpastes. Some toothpastes can dry out your lips. Tartar-control products are the most common irritants to your lips. Switching to a baking soda formula can solve the problem, says John E. Wolf, M.D., chairman of the Department of Dermatology at Baylor College of Medicine in Houston.

Nose around for a solution. It's −10° outside, and there's no lip balm to be found. No problem. Just try this: Rub your finger along the side of your nose, then rub it around your lips. Your finger will pick up a little of the oil that's naturally on your nose, the kind the lips are looking for.

Of course, you risk social embarrassment if someone catches a side view of you in the act and gets the wrong idea about your finger-to-nose-to-mouth move. But, hey, life is full of risks. And the truth will be on your lips.

Drink up. Drinking additional fluids in the winter is a natural and easy way to keep your lips from chapping. As you get older, your cells' ability to retain moisture decreases. So try to drink a glass of water every two hours, and humidify the air in your home and office.

Coughing

- Coughing keeps you awake at night
- Your coughing annoys other people

What It ⁇ Means

Most people cough at least once or twice an hour. It's a natural reflex that clears the throat and helps keep irritants out of the lungs. But when coughing keeps you awake at night, grows so persistent that you are physically tired or becomes so annoying that no one can stand being around you, it's not normal.

Bouts of coughing are usually the result of an infection caused by a cold or flu. Coughs can also be caused by stomach acids creeping into the esophagus, by inhaling irritants such as cigarette smoke and by breathing cold, dry air.

Before treating your cough, you need to figure out whether you *should* treat it. There are two kinds of coughs. First there's a productive cough. That's the kind that brings up gooey phlegm so that you can spit it out. You want to get the phlegm out. So that kind of cough is a good cough. If it's possible, let it run its course.

A dry, hacking cough doesn't bring up phlegm. All it does is irritate your throat, making you cough some more.

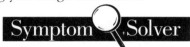

Symptom Solver

If you have a dry cough, here's how to muzzle it.

Take your medicine like a man. There are a number of over-the-counter cough suppressants that will quickly calm a dry, hacking cough. You don't need to root through name brands. According to the American Academy of Otolaryngology, the generic brands are just as effective. Just be sure that you get the right active ingredient.

Cough suppressants usually contain one of four ingredients: codeine, dextromethor-phan, diphenhydramine or guaifenesin. Codeine is great at suppressing coughs, but it also can upset the stomach and make you constipated. A suppressant containing dextromethorphan is probably the better choice. It suppresses the nerve signals that tell your body to cough, but without the side effects caused by codeine.

Diphenhydramine is an antihistamine that can treat coughs but also will make you drowsy. Guaifenesin is an expectorant that is supposed to loosen up mucus. Though approved by the Food and Drug Administration, clinical trials haven't proved its effectiveness. Drinking lots of fluids (water, juice, tea) will make your cough more productive, regardless of whether you are taking an expectorant.

Swallow a soothing potion. Swallowing a mixture of honey, lemon juice and ground red pepper can soothe a cough and sore throat, says Elson Haas, M.D., director of the Preventive Medical Center of Marin in San Rafael, California. The honey coats the throat, soothing the pain. The lemon is an astringent, which reduces inflammation and also clobbers germs with vitamin C. The ground red pepper brings circulation to the area, which speeds healing. It also is rich in vitamin A.

To make the potion, pour ¾ teaspoon of honey into a tablespoon and then fill the rest with lemon juice. Sprinkle the red pepper on top. You can take it four times a day, Dr. Haas says.

Put the men in menthol. Menthol, a common ingredient in some over-the-counter cough drops, is the principal component of the essential oil derived from peppermint. One study found that using menthol as a chest rub reduced coughs within 30 minutes.

Raise your head. If you usually cough only at night, you might be experiencing a condition called gastroesophageal reflux, in which stomach acids creep upward into the esophagus. The American Academy of Otolaryngology recommends elevating the head of your bed six to eight inches to keep the acids from creeping upstream.

Dizziness

- Problem balancing
- Possible spinning sensation

What It ? Means

When you read in the backseat of a moving car, your eyes tell the brain you're sitting still. But your ears feel the 55-mile-per-hour motion of the car. Your brain screams, "Yikes. Who's right?" And you feel queasy.

There are tons of things that can send conflicting messages to the brain and end up causing dizziness. And that's what makes dizziness so difficult to treat. Poor blood flow to the brain and to the ear is one common culprit in older patients. High blood cholesterol can reduce blood flow. So can stimulants such as nicotine and caffeine, as can an excessively salty diet.

Also, elderly people get dizzy more often because of degeneration to their inner ears, nerves and other parts of what's known as the vestibular system. Viral and bacterial infections in the ear can hamper nerve connections to the brain. Traumatic damage to parts of the ear can cause problems. And an accumulation of fluid in the ear can cause Ménière's disease, which results in a spinning sensation, ringing in the ears, ear pressure and hearing loss.

Symptom Solver

Because dizziness has so many causes, treating it can be a trial-and-error process. Here are a number of things to try, recommended by Brian W. Blakley, M.D., Ph.D., associate professor of otolaryngology at Wayne State University Medical Center in Detroit. But keep in mind that persistent or extreme dizziness problems should be treated with a doctor's care.

Lie still. When in the middle of a dizzy spell, keep your head as still as you can and lie down. Remain that way until you feel better. When you're ready to get up, first move your eyes, then your arms and legs and then the rest of your body—slowly.

Lend an ear. Exercises work especially well for people who have traumatic or degenerative damage to the ear, but not as well for people who have Ménière's disease, says Dr. Blakley. They help retrain your vestibular system. Here are a couple to try.

- Sit on the side of a bed. Do a side bend as far to the right as you can. Hold for 20 seconds. Sit up and then do the other side. Repeat three times on each side three or four times a day.
- Sit on the edge of a bed. Turn your head 45 degrees to the right and then lower the top of your head, moving your left ear toward your left knee. Return to the starting position and then do the same thing on the other side. Repeat as quickly as you can for 20 seconds three times a day.

Stash the saltshaker. Salt restriction may help some people with Ménière's disease because it may reduce the amount of fluid in the inner ear, says Herman Jenkins, M.D., chairman of the equilibrium subcommittee for the American Academy of Otolaryngology and professor of otorhinolaryngology at Baylor College of Medicine in Houston. That means keeping sodium intake to only two grams a day; that's less than a half-teaspoon of salt. Such a low-salt diet requires major food label reading because almost everything you eat contains sodium.

Try tai chi. Studies show that the ancient Chinese martial art tai chi can improve balance. The activity helps because it includes head-eye motions that can recalibrate the inner ear. In one study, people who took tai chi for two months improved their balance by about 10 percent. But not all tai chi is created equal. The best tai chi program would be one that is a joint approach between physical therapy and tai chi, says Timothy Hain, M.D., a neurologist at Northwestern University in Chicago and lead researcher of the study.

Ear Pain

- Earache

- Muffled hearing

- Sensation that there's pressure building up in the ear

What It ? Means

Ears are a lot like automatic cameras. If you accidentally spilled liquid laundry detergent all over the camera, the button would get gooped up. And you wouldn't be able to press it. Other parts would get gooped up and not move. And the camera wouldn't work.

That's sort of what happens when you get an earache, except usually there's no laundry detergent involved.

The most common type of earache occurs in children when the pus and mucus from a cold travel up the eustachian tube into the middle ear.

As you age, that type of earache occurs less often. That's because an infant's skull keeps the eustachian tube—which runs from the nose to the ear—short and flat. As you grow, the tube elongates, providing better functioning abilities, says Clough Shelton, M.D., associate professor of otolaryngology-head and neck surgery at the University of Utah in Salt Lake City.

However, it doesn't take pus—or even laundry detergent—to cause ear pain. A simple imbalance of air pressure on either side of the eardrum can muffle hearing and inflict pain. That's what happens when your ear hurts during an airplane flight.

Though adults don't tend to get middle-ear infections, they do get infections in the outer-ear canal. Commonly called swimmer's ear, the problem results from a buildup of moisture, which promotes bacteria growth in the canal leading to the eardrum.

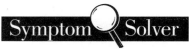
Symptom Solver

Once you have an ear infection, you'll need to see a doctor for antibiotic or antifungal treatment. But there are plenty of ways to prevent infections and ear pain.

Rub it out. There are various drops sold over the counter at the drugstore that help prevent swimmer's ear. But it's probably more convenient to look in your kitchen cabinet. White vinegar contains acetic acid, which is what is used in the swimmer's ear products, says John House, M.D., professor of otolaryngology at the University of Southern California School of Medicine in Los Angeles.

Placing a few drops of diluted white vinegar (50% water/50% vinegar) in each ear after swimming will dry the ear canal and help restore the natural acidity. Or you can use rubbing alcohol, which will dry and disinfect the ear. Sometimes, however, rubbing alcohol can sting, Dr. House warns.

Stay outside. The wax in your ears helps prevent bacterial growth. So when you consistently remove it with cotton swabs, you make yourself more prone to infection, says Dr. Shelton. Usually, wax will migrate to the outer ear all by itself. So the only cleaning you need to do is to just wipe off the opening of the ear (the part you can see) with a washcloth, he adds.

Swallow. When you're in an airplane, swallowing will open the eustachian tube that runs to your ear, pumping air behind the eardrum and equalizing the pressure, says Dr. Shelton. Yawning and chewing gum will create the same effect.

Decompress. When you're flying, take a decongestant that contains pseudoephedrine at least a half-hour before takeoff. The decongestant dilates the eustachian tube, making it easier to clear the ears of the air pressure that builds up inside. It also helps decrease secretions that may block the tube, says Jeffrey Jones, M.D., director of the Department of Emergency Medicine at Butterworth Hospital in Grand Rapids, Michigan.

Eye Discomfort

- Watery eyes
- Bloodshot eyes, but you haven't been near a bar in days
- Itchy eyes

What It Means

Tearing just might be one of the biggest tricks that your eyes can play on you. That's because one common cause of a watery eye is a dry eye.

Da-huh? That's what our reaction was when we asked Robert Abel, Jr., M.D., clinical professor of ophthalmology at Thomas Jefferson University in Philadelphia, to tell us why eyes water. He kept talking about dry eyes. We kept interrupting: "Now, doc. Don't mean to be rude, but we don't want to know about dry eyes. We want to know about watery eyes."

"That's what I'm telling you about," he said.

The liquid in the eyes comes in different forms. There are the gushy tears that spill down your face when you watch *Old Yeller*, chop onions or find out that your wife is sleeping with your best friend. These come from the lacrimal glands and are almost always in abundant supply. Then there are the tears that lubricate your eyeballs. They come from the accessory lacrimal gland. If there aren't enough tears in the accessory lacrimal gland, small dry spots form on the eyes. This irritation causes the main lacrimal gland to be stimulated, leaving you with watery eyes, according to Dr. Abel.

Another cause of watery eyes is allergies. Whether you're allergic to your pet cat, pollen or your wife's perfume, the immune system triggers the release of histamine, which is a chemical that causes the eyes to tear, itch and get bloodshot. Chemicals such as fiberglass and the chlorine in swimming pools can cause similar reactions.

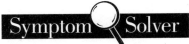

Symptom Solver

Before you can dry watery eyes, you have to know what's making them water in the first place. If it's allergies, you'll probably have other symptoms, like sneezing or a stuffy nose. If you suspect dry eyes, ask your ophthalmologist to perform a filter paper test. A piece of filter paper is placed on the eye for five minutes. Then the doctor measures how many tears your eye produced.

Whatever's causing your dry eyes, here are a few tips that can help.

Go fish. Dietary substances such as glucosamine sulfate, essential fatty acids and B vitamins will help keep your whole body, including the eyes, moist and lubricated. You can get these nutrients by eating more cold-water fish or using flaxseed oil. Or you can take supplements. "I take essential fatty acids once or twice a day. What I have found is that my skin is more moist. My eyes don't seem dry. And in the winter I don't get a dry cough," says Dr. Abel.

Don't rub. Really. Don't. "For five seconds it feels really good. And then it burns like hell," says Dr. Abel. The burning sensation that you experience comes from oil on your eyelid. When you rub the other side of the lid, you turn the oil into a thick, viscous tear film that burns.

Take a break. People who work at computers tend to get dry eyes. "When you do a lot of close work, you tend to stare. That dries out your eyes and makes them uncomfortable," says Dr. Abel.

Take an eye break every 20 minutes, advises James L. Cox, a behavioral optometrist in Bellflower, California. Look away from what you are doing and focus on something at least 15 feet away—across the room, down the hallway, out the window—to give your eyes a chance to rest.

Fever

• Your body temperature climbs above 99.9°F

What It Means

As far as the survival of the human race is concerned, a fever is always a good thing. But as far as your survival is concerned, a fever is only a good thing if it's a mild one.

Let's say that you have some horrible disease, like the Ebola virus. Despite what you may think, your body has already figured out that your days are pretty much numbered. And it knows that the stuff that's killing you is some pretty bad stuff. So your body decides to help out the rest of the human race by cranking up the heat so high that your brain dies and your heart can't function, keeping that vicious virus from getting inside someone else.

Good-bye, virus. Good-bye, you.

But let's say you have the flu. Your body assesses the situation and realizes that your immune system can easily fight off this virus. So your body temperature shoots up a few degrees. This isn't going to make your brain die or your heart stop. But it will rev up your white blood cells, cut off bodily processes that would otherwise feed the virus and slow down the virus's ability to reproduce.

Good-bye, virus. Hello again, you.

Symptom Solver

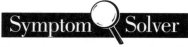

How you treat your fever largely depends on what your body is trying to tell you. Richard Honaker, M.D., of Carrollton, Texas, where he is president of Family Medicine Associates of Texas, says that you should see a doctor if:

• Your temperature keeps rising beyond 101°F. A fever of 106°F or higher is very dangerous.

• You are rapidly getting worse.
• Your fever has lasted more than three days.

If you only have a mild fever, however, the best thing to do is to grin and bear it. Various studies show that certain illnesses—including the flu and even chickenpox—last longer and are sometimes more severe when a fever is brought down with aspirin and other aids. When Los Angeles physician Michael Oppenheim, M.D., finds out that patients are worried about a mild fever, he advises them not to take their temperatures.

But that doesn't mean that you have to suffer silently. "Certainly if a fever is high enough that someone develops a severe headache or is in pain, it would be all right to use something to lower the fever," says Rex Daugherty, M.D., a physician in private practice in Pawhuska, Oklahoma.

Here are some proven techniques to beat the body heat.

Take two. Mom was right. The fastest way to bring down a fever is to take aspirin, acetaminophen or ibuprofen, says Dr. Daugherty. Follow the directions of the manufacturer. Avoid giving aspirin to a feverish child because of possible Reye's syndrome complications. Consider acetaminophen instead.

Cool it. Placing cool compresses on the head and neck can help reduce body temperature, Dr. Daugherty says.

Drink it away. Drinking iced beverages helps lower body fever, Dr. Daugherty says.

A fever will tend to dehydrate you, so it's important to drink plenty of liquids, says Gerald Rogan, M.D., a physician in Walnut Creek, California. Good choices include teas, juices, sports drinks and chicken and beef broths.

Sponge it off. Soak in tepid water and sponge the skin. "As the water evaporates off your body, it cools the skin and the blood vessels underneath it, which, in turn, may reduce your fever," says John C. Rogers, M.D., vice-chairman of the Department of Family Medicine at Baylor College of Medicine in Houston.

Forgetfulness

- You just met Joe (What's-his-name?)
- You can't remember what you ate for breakfast

What It ❓ Means

Grandpa can't find his car keys. Again. And once more, he starts fretting about "old-timer's" disease.

The fear of Alzheimer's is a common one, says Bruce K. Lowell, M.D., an internist and geriatrician in Queens, New York, and author of *Body Signals: When to Relax, When to Be Concerned and When to Go to the Doctor Immediately*. But in most cases, memory loss isn't anything to worry about. "It's very common to forget people's names. It's very common to forget things. It's very common to forget where you put your keys. You have a problem when you forget what you are supposed to do with the keys," says Dr. Lowell.

Some forgetfulness is a natural part of the aging process. The brain gradually loses its effectiveness when it comes to relaying signals and processing information. Such loss of brain function simply means that you need to put a bit more effort into remembering things.

Symptom 🔍 Solver

If you suspect that you or someone you know has Alzheimer's disease, a doctor's care is the best option. But for normal age-related memory problems, the following tips may help.

Lower that blood pressure. Studies show that high blood pressure during midlife can lead to memory problems later on. One study found that every ten-point increase in systolic blood pressure means more loss of cognitive skills later. If you don't know what your blood pressure is, it's time for a checkup.

Go for ginkgo. This herb can increase blood circulation to the brain, helping reverse short-term memory loss caused by poor circulation, says Varro E. Tyler, Ph.D., professor of pharmacognosy at Purdue University School of Pharmacy in West Lafayette, Indiana. Look for a product that contains 24 percent flavonoids and 6 percent ginkgolides. And follow the directions on the label, Dr. Tyler says.

Sleep on it. If you really want to remember something, think about it before going to sleep at night. Dreaming can help you hold on to new information, say researchers at Israel Weizmann Institute of Science in Rehovot, Israel. First, the sleep helps the brain consolidate information. Also, the body's natural circadian rhythms help the brain retain new information during sleep.

Repeat, for Pete's sake. A helpful trick for remembering the name of someone you just met is to repeat it a few times silently, waiting an extra second each time you repeat it, until there are four or five seconds between repetitions. "If you say a name quickly, it never enters your conscious mind," says Douglas J. Herrmann, Ph.D., a memory expert at the University of Maryland in College Park.

Be consistent. If you always put your car keys on the hook by the door, you'll never have to remember where they are. The same goes for other easily lost items such as umbrellas, wallets, watches and so forth. Set aside a special spot for them so that you don't need to trace your movements from the day before, says Joan Minninger, Ph.D., a psychotherapist in San Francisco and author of *Total Recall*.

Eat produce. If your intake of boron falls below one milligram a day, memory may suffer. Fruits and vegetables are prime sources of boron. To increase your boron intake, eat plenty of apples, grapes and broccoli. Drinking wine and sprinkling cinnamon on your food can also help, says James G. Penland, Ph.D., research psychologist at the U.S. Department of Agriculture Human Nutrition Research Center in Grand Forks, North Dakota.

Hair Loss

• No matter how long you put off getting it cut, your hair never gets in your eyes

What It ? Means

You can't remember ever seeing hair on top of your dad's head. And your older brother is already parting his hair closer and closer to his ear in a futile attempt to hide the lack of hair in the middle.

Are you next?

Only your genes know for sure, says Ken Hashimoto, M.D., professor and chairman of the Wayne State University School of Medicine in Detroit.

Although baldness is occasionally caused by outside factors such as ringworm, fungal infection, stress or medications, most of the time you can blame your parents. Male-pattern baldness—a receding hairline and/or a bald spot on the back of the head—runs in families. In fact, it comes from a gene that also makes you more sensitive to the hormone testosterone. In balding men, doctors believe, testosterone somehow damages the scalp's hair follicles, turning off their ability to sprout hair. At the same time, of course, this male hormone causes hair growth elsewhere on the body, like on the face, legs and chest.

You can inherit the tendency to lose hair from either parent. Just because your dad has a full head of hair doesn't mean that you're safe. You have to check out his dad, his dad's dad, your mom's dad and your mom's dad's dad. Well, you get the idea.

"If everyone in your family dies at the age of 80 with a beautiful head of hair, then you probably don't have to worry about it," says Dr. Hashimoto.

So if your dad's bald and your older brother's bald, will you go bald? You might. You might not. It really just depends on whether you inherited that bald gene, he says.

About 5 percent of men start losing hair in their twenties. By age 70, 80 percent of men are sporting shiny scalps (though some of those scalps are hidden underneath fake hair). The earlier you start balding, the more rapidly you're likely to lose your hair, Dr. Hashimoto says.

More is at stake than a cold pate. Research suggests that early balding may be linked to a higher risk of heart disease. Doctors have various explanations for the marriage between baldness and heart disease. If, as many experts suspect, bald men are sensitive to testosterone, this could make them more susceptible to heart disease. It's also possible that bald men have low levels of a compound called nitric oxide, which helps regulate blood pressure levels.

This is why, if your hair starts falling out during your twenties, it's particularly important to steer clear of other heart disease risk factors such as obesity, smoking, lack of exercise and high cholesterol.

Here's another reason to keep tabs on your heart health. Evidence suggests that a high-fat diet can be bad for your hair. It increases the amount of oil surrounding your hair follicles, which may mean more hair loss, says Dominic A. Brandy, M.D., in his book *A New Headstart!*

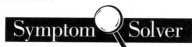 Symptom Solver

Among bald-headed men there's a popular saying: "Baldness is mind over matter—it really doesn't matter if the person doesn't mind."

Some men mind a lot and are willing to spend thousands of dollars keeping their heads under wraps, using medications, hair transplants and other types of cover-ups.

If you elect to have transplant surgery, a dermatologist will remove small patches of hair-sprouting scalp from the side of the head and reattach it to the non-hair-sprouting top. The problem is that you may continue to lose hair on parts of the "original" scalp. Then you would have to come in for a second transplant years later, says Dr. Hashimoto.

Drug treatment involves rubbing a medicated cream called minoxidil (Rogaine) onto your scalp twice a day—forever. The drug is available over the counter and costs about $25 for a month's supply, depending on the dose. The treatment can halt hair loss and sometimes spur hair growth. But once you stop using the stuff, your hair starts falling out all over again, Dr. Hashimoto says.

Then there are hairpieces. Good ones cost a lot. If you don't want everyone to know that you're wearing a rug, plan on spending at least $1,000. Of course, merely having lots of money isn't always the answer. Just look at Burt Reynolds.

There are plenty of things that you can do to optimize your bald look. Here's what the head experts advise.

Put away the comb. It's hard to resist. You know that it makes you look worse. But you do it anyway: Comb the hair on the side of your head over the top.

Listen to advice from Gillian Shaw, senior barber at Vidal Sassoon Salon in New York City: Don't do it. "From the front it might look pretty good, but from the back it looks pretty dreadful. It looks like Shredded Wheat on top of your head."

Keep it short. As hair falls out, there's a powerful tendency to compensate by letting the remaining hair grow. Don't, Shaw advises. "Something that's cut closer to the head makes the hair look a lot denser," she says. "You're really looking at a maintenance of cutting every four to five weeks with thinning hair. It requires a lot more cutting than with normal hair."

Keep it clean. Don't be afraid to wash your hair. It won't make it fall out faster. Neither will brushing it. In fact, washing your hair daily will give it the pick-me-up it needs to look

Bald—And Proud of It

It was 20 years ago, and Calvin Wellons was in his mid-forties. He was about 70 percent bald, and he wanted to look younger. Besides, he had just moved to a new town and figured that no one would know the difference. So he began wearing a hairpiece.

In those days, hairpieces were cumbersome. Wellons, a real estate developer in Morehead City, North Carolina, usually only put it on for special occasions.

"I was sitting at a dinner table one night, and when I reached over, it fell in another person's plate. This lady looked down at her food. I looked down at her food, and there sat that thing, turned upside-down. The lady then screamed out, it was most embarrassing. I never put it back on," recalls Wellons.

It's a story that gladdens the heart of his friend, John Capps III, also of Morehead City, who is the founder of a support group for bald men called Bald-Headed Men of America. His credo: "The Lord created only a few perfect heads, and the rest he covered with hair."

Before looking into the various options for covering up baldness, Capps urges men to consider whether it's really the lack of hair that's bothering them, or other, larger issues.

For more information, write to Bald-Headed Men of America, 102 Bald Drive, Morehead City, NC 28557.

fuller, Shaw says. Use a mild shampoo and conditioner to keep your hair from drying out.

Style it. Instead of jumping out of the shower, toweling off and getting on your way, stop and style your hair. Use a hair dryer. Make sure to use a low setting—you don't want to burn your scalp. Use a vent brush (the kind with holes in it) or a wide-toothed comb. And use the dryer to direct your hair, Shaw says.

Headaches: Tension-Type

• Pressing, tight feeling all around the head

• Jaw discomfort, neck pain and tender spots

What It Means

If you get headaches, chances are that these are the kind you get. Tension headaches cause a dull pain that makes your head feel like an overworked muscle. It's the most common kind of headache, affecting about 69 percent of men at some time during their lives.

Most tension headaches are caused by muscle tension around the temples and the back of your neck, says Frederick Freitag, D.O., associate director of the Diamond Headache Clinic in Chicago. They can also be caused by poor posture, medical problems such as arthritis or even depression.

Some people—about 10 percent of tension-headache sufferers—get chronic headaches that may occur nearly every day. For them, over-the-counter pain remedies are often ineffective.

Though tension-type headaches and migraines are very different—migraines are more severe and generally attack only one side of the head—there's generally an overlap. People who get migraines also get tension headaches and vice versa, says Dr. Freitag.

Symptom Solver

When you feel a headache coming on, the first thing you probably do is open the medicine cabinet and reach for a painkiller like aspirin or ibuprofen. Certain brands of

painkillers also contain caffeine. Avoid these. While caffeine may work great for a migraine headache, it actually makes a tension headache worse, says Marvin Hoffert, M.D., a headache specialist in private practice in Boston.

While any over-the-counter painkiller can help ease tension headaches, you might want to make ibuprofen your first choice, says Dr. Hoffert. People respond differently to different medications, so check with your doctor first. According to one study, 400 milligrams of ibuprofen is more effective than 650 milligrams of aspirin.

Here are some other things to try.

Stretch. Since tension headaches are often caused by muscle tension, stretching out those muscles can help ease the pain. For instance, if the back of your neck is tight, do slow neck stretches by holding your chin close to your chest, says Dr. Hoffert. You don't have to wait until the headache strikes. Throughout the day, periodically stretching the muscles that cause you pain can help prevent headaches from occurring.

If you can't quite tell where the tight spots are, a doctor can perform tests that pinpoint which muscles are stressed and then design an exercise and stretching program for you, says Dr. Hoffert. But we'll give you a hint. The areas usually affected are at the temples and the back of the neck.

Ice it. Putting an ice pack on the part of your head that hurts can be as effective as taking aspirin. "If they can get to the headache when it's a dull throb, close to 80 percent of people can abort their headaches," says Fred Sheftell, M.D., director of the New England Center for Headache in Stamford, Connecticut. Cold reduces inflammation of the blood vessels that often causes the pain.

Massage it. Rub the tiny ridge between your neck and the back of your head, right behind the ear lobes, for 10 to 15 minutes, says Dr. Sheftell. Then rub your temples and the back of the neck where your neck and shoulders meet. These are all prime tight-muscle spots, and a thorough massage can help them relax and ease the pain.

Watch what you eat. Some tension headaches are triggered by ingredients in food, like the MSG (monosodium glutamate) found in many processed foods, the nitrates in lunchmeat and the aspartame in diet sodas, says Dr. Freitag. The next time a headache strikes, think about what you ate just before. If you're able to identify a food that seems to be responsible, try avoiding it for a few weeks to see if things improve.

Sleep on schedule. Fluctuations in your normal sleep schedule— staying up all night, for example, followed by a day in bed—can trigger tension headaches. Try to keep regular hours, says Dr. Freitag.

Go easy on painkillers. If you find yourself using painkillers daily for headaches, you might be doing yourself more harm than good, cautions Dr. Hoffert. Painkillers are somewhat addictive, especially those that contain caffeine. So, eventually, they will work less effectively and actually cause more headaches to occur. If you're taking medications often to control headaches, check with your doctor.

Tune in. The best way to beat tension headaches is to listen to your body—to catch your tension and relax before the pain begins. "As you become aware of how your body talks to you, you get sophisticated enough to hear it whisper," says Joseph Primavera III, Ph.D., co-director of the Comprehensive Headache Center at Germantown Hospital and Medical Center in Philadelphia. "Then you can address the signs early on, and your body will never have to shout."

Research suggests that stopping to relax—even for as little as five minutes—at the first sign of pain may be enough to stop a headache before it gets started.

Hanging Up on Hangovers

You feel like the dung heap at the bottom of your parrot's cage. You make resolution Number 999 to never, ever drink again. Then you go back to sleep.

You don't need us to tell you that you shouldn't have guzzled that extra six-pack of beer. But maybe you could use a few pointers in the art of hangover warfare.

Rule one: Before going to bed after a night of carousing, eat some honey on toast and wash it down with a glass of water. The honey is loaded with fructose, which helps metabolize alcohol in your bloodstream, according to the National Headache Foundation. The water will help prevent dehydration, which leads to hangover. "Drink as much water as you can comfortably handle," says John Brick, Ph.D., executive director of Intoxikon International, a company in Yardley, Pennsylvania, that conducts alcohol and drug studies.

Rule two: Have bananas for breakfast. Drinking depletes the body of serotonin, a relaxing chemical produced in the brain. Bananas contain nutrients that help replenish the brain's natural serotonin stores.

Rule three: Take a painkiller in the morning. Forget taking it before bed to ward off tomorrow's headache. Acetaminophen, aspirin and other painkillers are designed to squelch pain when it hits. There's no proof that they will work ahead of time, says Dr. Brick.

Wash the dishes. Doing mundane tasks is a great way to relax. That's because you don't have to think about what you're doing. "Nothing induces a trance quicker than a boring kind of job, like doing the dishes. You do the dishes, you drift into thinking about something else; all of a sudden the dishes are done, and you snap out of it," says Dr. Primavera.

Take small breaks. "In the real world, maybe taking a deep breath, doing a stretch and staring out the window for a few minutes is all that you're going to get. Luckily, that's often just enough to keep you from triggering a headache," says Dr. Primavera.

Headaches: Migraine

- Aching pain on one side of the head

- Pain accompanied by other symptoms: nausea, dizziness, vomiting, numbness on one side of the face, cold hands

- Visual changes just before the pain: colors, shimmering lights, dark spots

- Pain lasting from a few hours to more than a day

What It Means

Migraine. Even the word sounds painful. But a migraine, most often an inherited condition that strikes women three times more often than men, is about more than just pain. About 40 percent of sufferers experience what is called the migraine aura. About 10 to 30 minutes before the pain starts, they may see flashing lights, wavy lines, dark spots, color splashes and other visual changes.

Then the pain sets in. It usually throbs on one side of the head, keeping pace with the beating of the heart. And it is usually accompanied by muscle tenderness, nausea and sensitivity to light and sound.

Doctors are not exactly sure what causes migraines. It may be that a decrease in the brain chemical serotonin causes blood vessels to expand and press on nearby nerves. Another theory centers on the ability of nerves in the brain to control the flow of potassium ions. In migraine sufferers, "triggers" such as food, weather conditions and sleep may hamper the nerves' ability to regulate the flow of potassium into the brain.

When too much potassium leaks out, the nerves release other chemicals to compensate. This, in turn, can make the nerves painfully sensitive. The pain is magnified when blood vessels in the brain, which naturally contract and expand, put additional pressure on the nerves. It's like getting a slap on your sunburned back.

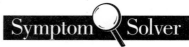

The first line of defense for any headache is over-the-counter pain medication. If you've already gone that route unsuccessfully, you might want to check the label. While aspirin, acetaminophen and ibuprofen are all effective at treating a migraine, it's best to use a product that also includes caffeine, since this makes the painkiller more effective, says headache specialist Dr. Marvin Hoffert.

"Be careful though," cautions Dr. Hoffert. "Some people are so sensitive to caffeine that its withdrawal can actually precipitate migraine headaches."

In addition to taking painkillers, here are some other tips you may want to try.

Be a magnesium magnet. One study found that about 42 percent of people suffering from intermittent migraines had low magnesium levels. Researchers suspect that magnesium may help regulate the swelling of blood vessels in the head that can contribute to migraine pain. Doctors aren't yet sure what the optimal magnesium dose is.

"I would tell people to eat as much as possible of dried beans, whole-grain foods, fish, nuts and seeds to achieve higher levels of magnesium without adding supplements," says study co-author Burton M. Altura, M.D., professor of physiology and medicine at State University of New York Health Science Center at Brooklyn College of Medicine.

Pull the trigger. Diet plays a role in 40 percent of migraine patients, says Dr. Frederick Freitag of the Diamond Headache Clinic. Items that can trigger migraines include chocolate, ripened cheese, alcohol, MSG (monosodium glutamate), citrus fruit, chicken liver and the preservatives in smoked or processed meat. Too much caffeinated cola or coffee can also trigger migraines, as can missing meals.

Be a regular guy. "Migraine sufferers do better if their lives are very orderly," says Dr. Freitag. That means going to bed and waking up at the same times every day. And it means eating at the same times every day.

See like a gremlin. Remember those cute, furry creatures in the movie *Gremlins?* They hated bright light. It could be that it gave them migraines. "Lighting conditions, from bright sunlight to fluorescent lighting, can play a strong role in migraines," says Dr. Freitag. He recommends wearing sunglasses outdoors and tinted lenses indoors, putting an antiglare screen on your computer monitor and using daylight-spectrum fluorescent bulbs.

Release endorphins. According to acupressurists, there are points all over the body that help relieve pain. The easiest one to find is located in the web of skin between the thumb and index finger. Pinch there and wait. The theory is that pain will encourage the body to release its natural painkilling endorphins, says Dr. Freitag.

Get help. A doctor can prescribe medication to ease migraine pain. There are two types of drugs to choose from. One type—called abortive—will alleviate pain after the migraine starts. The drug sumatriptan (Imitrex) is an abortive drug. Anyone getting prescription medication should start with this type of drug, says Dr. Freitag. People who get frequent headaches—more than two a month—may need preventive medication. Some of the same drugs used to treat high blood pressure, like propranolol (Inderal), will also help prevent migraines, says Dr. Freitag.

Nap Migraines in the Bud

It's a good excuse to give your boss when he finds you nodding off on the job. Sleep. Doctor's orders.

"Most people with a migraine, if they can get several hours of sleep, can stop the headache," says Dr. Frederick Freitag of the Diamond Headache Clinic.

Indeed, research suggests that in some cases taking a nap may be just as good as taking a pill.

Experts agree that medications that abort a headache (that is, cut an attack short) or painkillers remain the first line of defense. "But if you haven't aborted it, and you wind up with a full-blown attack, sleep is very helpful," says Seymour Diamond, M.D., of Chicago, executive director of the National Headache Foundation. It might actually reduce your need for migraine medication, he adds. One study suggested that people with mild migraines (with no accompanying nausea or vomiting) found relief with sleep and rest alone or were able to delay taking migraine medications when they napped.

Scheduling extra nap time won't help prevent migraines—it might actually provoke them. Try sleep and rest only if you're unable to block your migraine.

Write it down. Since migraines can be triggered by a variety of factors—not just food and sleep schedules but also such things as weather and stress—it's important to identify the main culprits. You should keep a headache diary, says Dr. Freitag. When you get a headache, write down everything you ate and drank for the past 24 hours. Then record what type of stress you have experienced, the weather and anything else that may have caused the headache. Eventually, you'll see a pattern and will have some idea of what to avoid in the future, he says.

Headaches: Cluster

• You have severe pain behind one eye

• Headaches occur in clusters or groups for periods of several weeks, then go into remission for several months

• Eyes tear and nose runs

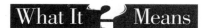

What It Means

Maybe we have that Oedipus story all wrong.

It could be that the day he figured out he had murdered his father and married his mother, Oedipus took the news well. He could accept his fate. But what he couldn't handle was a sudden cluster headache that felt like someone was sticking a hot poker in his eye.

Maybe, just maybe, Oedipus thought that gouging out his eyes would stop the horrible pain.

Hey, it's possible.

Anyway, the point is that cluster headaches are the ultimate in pain. They're so bad that some victims liken the agony to having an eye pulled out. For some, the pain is so severe that they commit suicide.

The pain, which often strikes at night, lasts about 45 minutes and is usually centered behind one eye. On the side of the head with the pain, the eye may tear and the nose get congested. Worse, the attacks usually come in waves, lasting for days, weeks or even months, and then disappear for several months or more.

Cluster headaches are rare but are five times more common in men than women. There's still speculation about what causes them. One theory centers on an excess of activity in the nervous system that makes some of the

nerves in the head more sensitive than usual. When the arteries in the head narrow and expand—as they normally do—those sensitive nerves start screaming. The attacks also may be caused by a problem in the body's biological clock: Cluster headaches tend to strike within a few weeks of the longest and shortest days of the year and also when clocks are changed at the beginning and end of daylight savings time.

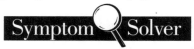

Not only are cluster headaches painful but they are also difficult to treat without the help of a doctor. But with a doctor's care, cluster patients do fairly well. Though there are only a handful of medications for treating the ailment, they tend to be very effective, says headache specialist Dr. Marvin Hoffert.

Other than taking prescription medication, here are a few things that you can do to stop the pain.

Inhale. Inhaling pure oxygen through a face mask can relieve cluster headache pain in five to ten minutes, says Dr. Hoffert. It's particularly effective in those ages 50 years and younger. You can buy pure oxygen without a doctor's prescription, but Dr. Hoffert cautions that you should talk to your doctor first about whether you may benefit from using oxygen.

Beware of the sin tax. Men who get cluster headaches are often heavy drinkers and smokers who have type A personalities, according to one study. And alcohol can trigger a headache within minutes during a susceptible period, says Dr. Frederick Freitag of the Diamond Headache Clinic. For some people, cutting out alcohol, nicotine and stress can help prevent the headaches, Dr. Freitag says.

Pound the pavement. It may be the last thing you feel like doing, but exercise can abort cluster headaches, says Dr. Freitag. "It sounds like a silly thing to do for a headache. But if cluster sufferers can really get their hearts pumping, it can actually help stop their attacks," he says.

Jaw Pain

- You hear a clicking noise when you open your mouth

- Your jaw hurts

- The pain spreads, causing muscle aches in the neck or headache

What It Means

You can use it as a stupid party trick. You open your mouth wide: "Pop." For a second, everyone's drinks are suspended in midair as they wonder how you accomplished that sound merely by opening your mouth.

The problem is that it won't earn you a spot on *The Late Show with David Letterman.* Plus, that pop is often followed by "ouch."

A popping, aching jaw may be a sign of temporomandibular disorder. That's TMD for short, and it that means that you have something wrong with the temporomandibular joint that hinges your jaw to your skull.

You can injure the joint in a number of ways. Grinding your teeth is a common culprit. Physical injury, like getting whacked in the face, can also do it. If you're under a lot of stress, bad habits such as gritting your teeth and chewing on pens can put painful pressure on the joint.

Once injured, the hinge loses its alignment and doesn't provide a friction-free ride as your jaw opens and closes. Instead, it allows bone to rub against bone, creating a clicking sound.

Clicking is usually the first sign of trouble. If the jaw abuse continues, the joint can erode. In some people the jaw will lock every once in a while. Eventually, it may get so bad that you won't be able to completely open your mouth, says Brendan Stack, D.D.S., director of the National Capitol Center for Craniofacial Pain in Vienna, Virginia.

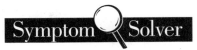

Symptom Solver

If you have a click in your jaw but no pain, you might not need to do anything. "If it doesn't hurt, don't fix it," says Dr. Charles H. Perle of the Academy of General Dentistry and the American Dental Association.

But it's still a good idea to have your dentist check it out to determine the cause, adds Dr. Cherilyn G. Sheets of the Academy of General Dentistry. If it turns out that there's something seriously wrong, you'll want to catch it early.

A painful jaw, however, always demands attention. Of course, taking an anti-inflammatory painkiller such as aspirin or ibuprofen should quickly help ease the pain. But here are some less obvious ways to get relief.

Take a jaw break. While the joint is hurting, eat only soft, mushy foods, such as applesauce, soup and oatmeal. And avoid chewing gum, says Dr. Sheets.

Also avoid chomping nonfood items like pen caps, says Harold T. Perry, D.D.S., Ph.D., professor emeritus of orthodontics at Northwestern University Dental School in Chicago.

Compress it. You can soothe the jaw by wrapping ice in a towel and applying it for ten minutes, Dr. Sheets says. Take a ten-minute break, then repeat the ice application.

Say mmmmm. Be conscious of your jaw's normal resting position. When you feel yourself tensing up your facial muscles, try to relax, says Dr. Perle. He recommends putting your lips together but keeping your teeth apart.

Keep a lid on it. To avoid inflicting unnecessary pain on yourself, try to keep from opening your mouth wide when yawning or laughing, says Dr. Perle.

Stop the grind. People who grind their teeth at night often suffer from jaw pain. If you're a snoozing grinder, ask your dentist to fit you with a night-guard mouthpiece. It won't stop the grinding, but it will protect your teeth and act as a shock absorber, says Dr. Sheets.

Nosebleed

• You feel like you're auditioning for a *Rocky* sequel

• Blood trickles out of your nose or down the back of your throat

What It Means

That nose is one fragile piece of equipment.

It's lined with hundreds of tiny blood vessels that are close to the skin's surface. And the inner lining takes a lot of abuse. Think of all the blasts it gets when you rear back and blow that honker. And think of all that nasal probing that goes on, especially when no one else is around.

When you take a minute to put yourself in your nostrils' place, you can't help but feel a bit proud for holding off as many bleeds as you do.

Nosebleeds come in two forms. The one we're most familiar with is called the anterior nosebleed. The blood oozes down from the front part of the nose and out the nostrils. Anterior nosebleeds are common in dry climates or during the winter months, when the dry air parches the nasal membranes until they crust, crack and bleed.

The other kind of nosebleed, called the posterior bleed, is more serious. Blood gushes from deep within the nose and tends to run down the back of the mouth and throat. Often it's a result of injury, as when someone whacks you in the nose.

Symptom Solver

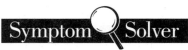

There are a variety of ways to stop a nosebleed. Here are some of our favorites.

Sit up. It's a natural reflex to want to tilt your head back or lie down. But it actually helps to sit up during a nosebleed because it reduces the blood pressure in the nasal area, says Rex Daugherty, M.D., a physician in private practice in Pawhuska, Oklahoma.

Pinch it. People do this intuitively, if only to keep blood from getting all over their clothes. Most of the blood that gushes out of your nose comes from the area inside the tip. So simply pinching your nostrils shut and holding them closed for at least 10 to 15 minutes should stop the bleeding, says Dr. Daugherty.

For best results, press toward your face while pinching. "Most people will pinch it for a little while. Then they'll relax pressure to see if it's still bleeding. Instinctively, then, they want to blow the nose to get the clots out. That starts the whole thing over again," says Dr. Daugherty.

Double-team and press. Acupressurists use strategic points on the body to relieve nosebleeds. A preferred location is just above the upper lip below the nose. Another is in the large hollow at the base of the skull. Use your fingers to press in both places simultaneously, says Michael Reed Gach, Ph.D., founder and director of the Acupressure Institute in Berkeley, California, and author of *Acupressure's Potent Points*.

Cool it. Putting an ice pack on your neck or cheek will cool blood flowing into the area and help promote clotting, says Dr. Daugherty.

Keep it protected. After a bleed, your nose is still sensitive. To prevent starting another gush, avoid blowing or picking it. Don't strain to pick things up, which can increase your blood pressure. And try to keep your head higher than your heart, advises Jack B. Anon, M.D., of Erie, Pennsylvania, chairman of the nasal and sinus committee for the American Academy of Otolaryngology-Head and Neck Surgery.

Seal it. For stubborn bleeds, the American Academy of Otolaryngology recommends four pumps from a decongestant spray up each nostril. This will shrink blood vessels and help reduce bleeding. Some decongestant sprays that can help include Afrin, Duration and Neo-Synephrine.

Straighten it out. If your nose has just been broken, fast action can help ensure that you don't go through life with a crooked sniffer, says Allan Levy, M.D., team physician for the New York Giants and co-author of *A Sports Injury Handbook*. Place the fingers of both hands on either side of your nose and force it into its normal position. Then get to a doctor right away.

Preventing Nosebleeds

If you get frequent nosebleeds, you should try the following techniques.

Blow carefully. You can make yourself prone to nosebleeds by blowing your nose too vigorously. That irritates the nose lining, forming scabs that eventually bleed. "One of the main things is not to stop up one side and blow out the other," says Dr. Daugherty.

Lube that sniffer. If your nose is dry, put lubricating cream or ointment the size of a pea on the end of a fingertip and rub it up inside the nose, especially on the middle portion. The American Academy of Otolaryngology recommends using over-the-counter lubricating creams like A and D ointment, Mentholatum, Vicks VapoRub or petroleum jelly. You should lube your nose at least once a day before bedtime, though some people may need to do it as frequently as three times a day.

Vaporize your world. Use a vaporizer or cool-mist humidifier to offset indoor dryness, especially in winter months, when the air tends to be drier, says Dr. Anon.

Be careful with alcohol. According to a study, regular alcohol consumption can cause frequent, more serious and more prolonged nosebleeds by reducing the blood's ability to clot and also by dilating the nose's blood vessels. If you're drinking a lot and also having regular nosebleeds, it may be time to cut back.

Advice from the Corner

One of the most taxing moments of Al Gavin's life occurred the night that Walter Sealy's nose went out of joint after his opponent rammed it with his head.

Gavin, then a fledgling cut man, knew that he had to stop the blood for the fight to continue. "We have an expression in my business: 'If you don't stop the flow, you go,' " says Gavin, who got the bleeding under control before the next round, enabling Sealy to go on to win the ten-round bout.

After that auspicious beginning in the 1960s, Gavin moved on to other noses and body parts. Today he's the cut man for heavyweight boxers Bruce Seldon and Riddick Bowe.

Here's what Gavin uses to stop nosebleeds fast.

Pressure. He uses his hands to put pressure on both sides of the bridge of the nose.

Ice. He puts it just below the point where he's squeezing.

Adrenaline. For serious bleeds, he puts some adrenaline on a cotton swab and puts it up the nose to shrink the blood vessels. (This is not something you want to try at home.)

Relaxation. "It's a mind-over-matter thing. If you tell the person to slow down and relax, he helps himself a lot," says Gavin.

Dodging. He advises pugilists to move their heads a lot so that they have less chance of coming in contact with an incoming fist.

Runny and/or Stuffy Nose

• Breathing through your nose is difficult

• You feel like you should own stock in Kleenex

What It Means

There are times when you want to cut off your nose to spite your cold or allergy.

Since you're reading this chapter, apparently this is one of those times. When you're congested, breathing through your nose is like sucking air through a collapsed straw. And upstairs, the mucous hose is running full blast.

That means that a virus, some bacteria or an allergen is trying to get up your nose. That stuff doesn't belong there. And it especially doesn't belong further inside your body. So the body's natural response is to trap invaders with mucus and evict them. That's why your nose runs. The mucus is carrying out pollen, virus and other invading particles.

Another defensive response is to make it difficult for invading particles to crawl farther inside the body. So thousands of tiny blood vessels in the nose expand, causing membranes to swell. That makes passageways smaller and also floods the area with germ-fighting white blood cells.

Sometimes your nose will only run. Other times it will only get stuffy. Sometimes you'll be cursed with both.

"When it comes to allergies, there are two kinds of people: the runners and the blockers," says Dr. Jack B. Anon of the American Academy of Otolaryngology-Head and Neck Surgery. "You tend to see a runny nose more with someone who has seasonal allergies in the spring and fall. A person who has chronic, year-round allergies tends to have more congestion."

Sometimes the stuffiness is compounded by a secondary infection. When the membranes in the nose swell up, the sinuses can't drain. And then you can get a bacterial infection on top of the allergy or viral infection. You'll know that you have a secondary infection because your mucus will turn yellow or green.

By the way, a mild amount of stuffiness is normal. On an average day, for instance, pay attention to how you breathe through your nose. You'll probably prefer either your right or left nostril. A few hours later, you'll find that you're using the opposite nostril. That's because one side or the other is naturally congested all the time. The body takes advantage of this feature, which permits various nose glands to function independently.

Symptom Solver

Here's what to do to make breathing a bit easier.

Stop and smell the rosemary. A traditional remedy for a stuffed-up nose is rosemary. You can buy the essential oil in health food stores. Either sniff the oil straight or put a few drops in a small pot of boiling water and then inhale the steam, says Jeanne Rose of San Francisco, president of the National Association for Holistic Aromatherapy in Boulder, Colorado, and author of *The Aromatherapy Book.*

Caution: Before inhaling, take the pot off the stove and let it cool so that no active boiling is taking place. (If the water is actively boiling, it can scald your face.) Hold your face about a foot away from the pot and cover your head and shoulders with a towel to trap the steam.

Wet your sniffer. Keeping the nasal lining moist will help prevent stuffiness caused by winter's arid air. It's a good idea to keep a humidifier running in your bedroom at night to moisten the air that you breathe, says Dr. Rex Daugherty of Pawhuska, Oklahoma.

Strip it. There are nasal strips available that can relieve nasal congestion and the snoring that accompanies it. The adhesive plastic strips cost about $5 at the drugstore. When taped across the bridge of your nose, they grab the skin over the flare of each nostril, opening the passageway. Studies show that the strips can reduce airway resistance by 31 percent.

Choose the right medicines. Antihistamines work best on congestion caused by allergies because they block the chemical (histamine) that causes the symptoms. They also help dry a runny nose. But cold and flu problems often call for decongestants, which work by shrinking swollen nasal passages, says Dr. Anon.

Spice it up. Eating spicy foods—seasoned with such high-octane ingredients as horseradish, mustard, ground red pepper, chili peppers or garlic—can temporarily blast open swollen passages.

Know how to blow. When you're congested, it may feel like you have a wad of gunk inside your nose. And you do. But it's not attached to anything. The stuffy feeling comes from swollen membranes. And you're not going to get it out of your nose no matter how hard you blow. So don't blast away or you might cause a nosebleed (see Nosebleed on page 50). Gently blow out without pinching your nostrils shut, says Dr. Daugherty.

Spray it yourself. Rather than using a powerful decongestant, you can make your own nasal spray by mixing ¼ teaspoon each of salt and baking soda in eight ounces of warm water, and then sniffing a handful every hour or so. This will help reduce congestion by clearing mucus and soothing inflamed membranes.

Hit the showers. Inhaling steam is probably the quickest drug-free way to break up congestion. So take a long, hot shower to open those nasal passages. That way, even you'll be able to tell that you smell better.

Drink up. Yet another reason to down the eight eight-ounce glasses of water experts advise you to drink each day: Water helps dilute mucus in your nose and sinuses and keeps it flowing freely.

Press for relief. Acupressure can help relieve the congestion caused by allergies and colds. Below are two techniques that you can try, recommended by Dr. Michael Reed Gach of the Acupressure Institute.

Acupressure Techniques

Welcoming Perfume: Use your middle finger to press just to the side of the nostril under the cheekbones with the pressure angled slightly up. At the same time, use your index finger to press the next point.

Facial Beauty: Press next to your index finger at the bottom of the cheekbone directly under the center of your eye.

Sneezing

• You're beginning to think your name is Gesundheit because that's all that people seem to say to you

What It ✏ Means

What is it about a simple sneeze that prompts all within earshot to verbally trip over one another with grand wishes of well-being? The ancient Greeks wished "long life" for sneezers. And if you sneeze in a crowd these days, you're likely to hear a chorus of "gesundheit," meaning good health.

Failure to sneeze, then, apparently condemns you to a short life and bad health, which seems rather odd, since sneezing is nothing more profound than having an irritated nose.

"Any nasal irritation may set off a sneeze," says Dr. Jack B. Anon of the American Academy of Otolaryngology-Head and Neck Surgery.

The list of sneeze stimulators seems endless. Some offenders are typical allergens such as pollen and dust, which the nose evicts with a forceful sneeze. But sneezing can also be stimulated by other, seemingly unrelated things, like sunlight, urination, shivering or sexual excitement. One small study suggests that some sneezing may be linked to our circadian rhythms, which may be why some people habitually sneeze at the same time every day.

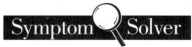

Symptom 🔍 Solver

Since most sneezes are simply your body's attempt to evict unwanted substances from the nasal passages, don't resist the urge. Let your body get rid of whatever it is. But be polite. If you have a cold, sneeze-blown droplets of mucus can travel as far as 12 feet. So cover your nose and mouth with a handkerchief or tissue, advises Dr. Rex Daugh-

erty of Pawhuska, Oklahoma.

Then try one of the following remedies to stop the sneeze in its tracks.

Apply pressure. There's an acupressure point between the nose and upper lip. You can abort a sneezing fit by firmly pressing the skin against the gum, says Dr. Michael Reed Gach of the Acupressure Institute and author of *Acupressure's Potent Points*. To find out more about using acupressure to relieve hay fever, call the Acupressure Institute at 1-800-442-2232.

Drink some coffee. Back in his hectic residency days, Vincent Tubiolo, M.D., discovered that the same coffee that woke him up in the morning also eased his hay fever. Now a fellow of allergy and immunology at Harbor-UCLA Medical Center in Torrance, California, Dr. Tubiolo has put coffee to the test. In one small study, he gave people with hay fever either 400 milligrams of caffeine—about the equivalent of three cups (six ounces each) of brewed coffee—or a placebo. Four hours later, those in the caffeine group noted a 51 percent reduction in hay fever symptoms, including sneezing, while those taking the placebo only experienced a 19 percent improvement. Larger studies still need to be done, but Dr. Tubiolo speculates that caffeine helps relieve hay fever symptoms by preventing inflammation in the nasal cavities.

Take an antihistamine. If you have allergies, over-the-counter medications like diphenhydramine (Benadryl) will block the body's production of the chemical (histamine) that can cause sneezing, says Dr. Anon. But be wary of taking over-the-counter antihistamines before going to work; they may cause drowsiness and lack of coordination. As an alternative, your doctor may prescribe nonsedating antihistamines like astemizole (Hismanal) and terfenadine (Seldane).

Wear shades. Experts aren't sure why, but in some people, generally men, sunlight triggers a bizarre series of nerve impulses that result in sneezing. There's an easy solution: Wear sunglasses when you go outside.

Snoring

- Your bedmate complains that sleeping with you is like sleeping in a train station

- Gasping or choking during sleep

- Excessive sleepiness during the day

What It Means

Women put on weight in their butts and thighs. Men put it on in the belly and neck. And that makes all the difference when it comes to snoring: Men do it louder and more often.

Excess neck fat is a major cause of snoring. The fat chokes off room for air to travel. Then, when you lie down at night, gravity pulls tissues in the mouth and throat downward, choking off still more room. With each breath, that hanging tissue vibrates. And your bed partner hears "Hhgzzzzz."

Though fat is a common cause of snoring, anything that narrows airways in the nose, mouth or throat—like an overbite, stuffy nose or enlarged tonsils—can have the same effect.

Snoring is more than merely a nuisance to your bedmate. Over time it can strain the heart, contributing to heart disease. Snorers also tend to develop high blood pressure at a younger age than nonsnorers.

Symptom Solver

In some cases home remedies are all that you'll need to silence a snore. But if you suspect that you have sleep apnea (see "When the Breathing Stops" on page 56), do yourself a favor and see your doctor.

Go natural first. There are a number of simple remedies that doctors say can help keep your airways open. Things that you may want to try include:

- Place bricks or blocks of wood under the two legs at the head of your bed, advises Edmund Pribitkin, M.D., an otolaryngologist at Thomas Jefferson University Hospital in Philadelphia. This will elevate your upper body slightly, reducing gravity's effect on your tongue and helping to keep airways open.

- Avoid alcohol, tranquilizers and antihistamines before bedtime, says Alex Clerk, M.D., director of the sleep disorders clinic at Stanford University. Each of these has effects that can make your muscles overly relaxed and contribute to snoring.

- Try decongestants or steroid nasal sprays to combat nasal congestion that might be contributing to snoring, Dr. Clerk says. Some people have had success using special adhesive strips (available over the counter at many drugstores), which you tape across the nose to help keep the passages open.

- Stay off your back. Sleeping on your back allows the tongue to fall backward into your throat, narrowing the airway. Some experts advise sewing a small pouch in the back of a T-shirt or pajama top and putting a tennis ball inside. The resulting bulge will help you resist the urge to roll over onto your back at night, even when you're asleep.

Whistle while you work. Research suggests that singing and whistling may help to tone the very muscles that want to fall forward when you sleep. By incorporating singing or whistling into your daily routine, you may help cut down on the cacaphony at night.

Skip the snack. Avoid nibbling three hours before retiring. The process of digestion causes muscles everywhere—including those in your throat—to loosen up.

Shed some pounds. People who snore and have sleep apnea tend to have a neck circumference of 17 inches or more—about the size of a supermodel's waist. Trimming down can cure snoring and sleep apnea in some people. At the very least, it can play an important role in any stop-snoring plan. "It's a good recommendation to lose weight because it will help make other treatments more effective," says Dr. Clerk.

Stop being a butt head. Studies show that smoking can aggravate snoring. The best thing you can do is quit entirely, but even cutting back may help.

Wear a retainer. A specially trained dentist or orthodontist can fit you with an oral appliance that will keep your tongue from falling backward into your throat, which can help reduce snoring, says John Ruddy, M.D., assistant clinical professor at the National Jewish Center/University of Colorado Health Sciences Center in Denver.

Use a mask. Wearing a pressurized mask when you sleep is perhaps the most effective way to treat snoring, says Dr. Clerk. This system, called continuous positive airway pressure, or CPAP, maintains the upper airway in an open position while you sleep.

The drawback is that wearing a mask at night can be cumbersome, inconvenient and, for some people, claustrophobic. It's a good idea to try as many different masks and machines as you can, since some are more comfortable than others, says Dr. Ruddy.

Consider surgery. For mild to moderate snoring problems, surgical treatment has come a long way, says Jack Coleman, M.D., of Nashville, chairman of the sleep disorders committee for the American Academy of Otolaryngology-Head and Neck Surgery. Today, a doctor can use a laser to vaporize excess tissue, which in some cases can eliminate snoring altogether. It's a simple outpatient procedure that's done with a local anesthetic. Some people, however, need multiple sessions over a six-month period, says Dr. Coleman.

When the Breathing Stops

If you're one of those guys with bed-shaking, wall-rattling snores, you could have a condition called sleep apnea, in which breathing frequently stops during sleep. That's the quiet part. Things get noisy when breathing resumes—often with gasps, snorts and snores.

In men with sleep apnea, the airway occasionally gets blocked during sleep. That means that the sleeper doesn't breathe until the airway opens up—which can be 10, 20, 60 seconds or even more. Even if the airway stays open, sometimes the actual drive to breathe shuts down. Either way, the result is oxygen deprivation. That's what causes the sleeper to awaken with snorts or snores.

You already know that snoring isn't good for your health. Sleep apnea is much worse. Because you take in too little oxygen, the heart works harder to pump the oxygen you do have through the body. Over time, that can lead to an irregular heartbeat, an enlarged heart and high blood pressure. And because people with sleep apnea don't sleep well at night, they're often exhausted during the day. Because they're constantly drowsy, they're nearly seven times more likely to get in car accidents than people without this condition. They also may experience problems with memory, thought and work performance.

If you suspect that you have sleep apnea, see a doctor right away. Many of the same strategies that can be used to relieve snoring will help improve this condition as well.

Sore Throat

- It hurts to swallow

- Your throat hurts even when you don't swallow

What It Means

At first it felt like the fast-food coffee you had this morning was way too hot. But after a while, it seemed more like a porcupine might have crawled down your throat and got stuck. (It could happen.)

Sorry, but it's nothing that exotic. You didn't swallow a porcupine. And you can't sue the fast-food joint over that cup of steaming hot java. (Better call the lawyer back, pronto. What a shame—he seemed *so* excited.) No, your throat hurts because there's an inflammation somewhere between the back of your tongue and your voice box.

Viral and bacterial infections are usually the culprits. But allergies also can irritate the throat. And during the winter months, you can get a mild sore throat from breathing dry air, especially if a stuffy nose causes you to breathe through your mouth.

Symptom Solver

If you suspect that you have a bacterial infection such as strep throat (it will really hurt), see a doctor for antibiotic treatment. But if the cause is nonbacterial, such as a virus, cold or allergy, you'll need to ease the pain and help your immune system fight the infection. Here's how to do it.

Chase some vampires. Eat a clove of raw garlic twice a day. It will boost your immune system's ability to fight off the infection, says Dr. Elson Haas, director of the Preventive Medical Center of Marin. Or you can take odorless garlic capsules or tablets

purchased at health food stores. They are effective, but not as effective as the real thing.

Taste the ocean. "There's nothing much better than gargling with warm salt water," says Jack M. Gwaltney, M.D., chief of epidemiology and virology at the University of Virginia School of Medicine in Charlottesville.

Use 1½ teaspoons salt to one quart warm water for best results, advises Edward Mortimer, M.D., a pediatrician and epidemiologist at Case Western Reserve University in Cleveland.

Treat it gingerly. Ginger increases the body's circulation and induces sweating. Both aspects help cleanse the body and promote healing, says Dr. Haas. You can eat real ginger, drink it in tea or take a capsule. All three forms are available at health food stores.

Make your own potion. Swallowing a mixture of honey, lemon juice and ground red pepper can soothe a sore throat, says Dr. Haas. The honey coats the throat, nurturing away the pain. The lemon is an astringent, which reduces inflammation and also clobbers invaders with vitamin C. The ground red pepper brings circulation to the area, which speeds healing. It also is rich in vitamin A. Pour ¾ teaspoon of honey into a tablespoon and then fill it up the rest of the way with lemon juice. Sprinkle the red pepper on top. You can take it four times a day.

Feed your sweet tooth. Really. The sugar will soothe the pain. "Suck on something sweet," says Dr. Rex Daugherty of Pawhuska, Oklahoma. "I think a lot of the inexpensive, routine things such as hard candy and lemon drops are in a lot of respects much better than the expensive lozenges with menthol and local anesthetics. The more expensive lozenges do relieve the pain. But they leave your mouth dry. Plain hard candy is probably the best because it keeps the mouth moist."

Drink more. You'll want to keep your throat lubricated by drinking plenty of liquids. The American Academy of Otolaryngology suggests the old-time home remedy of warm tea with honey to soothe the throat.

Swollen Glands

- It hurts to swallow
- The usually pebble-size neck glands are large, hard and tender

What It Means

Think of the hundreds of lymph nodes scattered throughout your body as neighborhood firehouses. Most of the time, things are pretty quiet. Just a bunch of white blood cells, hanging around the station all day, playing cards and keeping the place spick-and-span.

But when a "fire" breaks out in your body, in the form of an infection, more white blood cells respond to the alarm, flooding into your nodes—commonly called glands—to extinguish the threat.

Usually, the nodes are soft, rubbery, movable masses of less than a quarter-inch in diameter. Their main responsibility is to remove toxins and other unwanted materials from the body.

But when the alarm sounds to fight an infection, they swell, becoming hard and tender as white blood cells rush in from your bone marrow and thymus gland.

In addition, your glands become the clearinghouse for germs that are dragged in from the front lines, digested and then disposed of.

There are more than 500 lymph nodes scattered throughout your body in places such as the neck, groin and armpits. You usually notice swollen glands in the neck, where more than 30 percent of your lymph nodes reside. But other glands in the body swell when there is an infection in the neighborhood. For instance, an infected leg sore will make the glands in the groin swell.

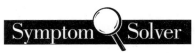

There's not much you can do for the glands themselves other than soothing them with a heating pad or warm washcloth for 15 minutes four times a day. What you need to do is concentrate on getting rid of the infection that is causing the glands to swell, says Dr. Rex Daugherty of Pawhuska, Oklahoma. You can do that by boosting your immune system's ability to fight. Just remember, some infections will need a doctor's care. If the glands remain swollen for more than a few days or are accompanied by fever, sore throat and other symptoms, you should check with your physician.

Make a cup of tea. Ginger increases your body's circulation and induces sweating. Both aspects help cleanse the body and promote healing, says Dr. Elson Haas of the Preventive Medical Center of Marin. If your glands are so swollen that you are having trouble swallowing, taking the ginger in tea form would be easiest. You can buy ginger tea at most health food stores.

Have some garlic. Garlic has natural antibiotic qualities. Eating a few cloves a day will help stimulate your body's immune system to kill off whatever infection is causing your glands to swell, says Dr. Haas. Eating it fresh probably has the strongest effect, he says. But you also can take it in odorless garlic capsule or tablet form.

Go for Echinacea. This herb can help rid the blood and lymph glands of toxic substances, Dr. Haas says. It's sold at most health food stores. In capsule form, take one or two twice a day at the onset of your symptoms.

Make it goldenseal. This herb can stimulate your liver, which helps clear up infection. It also strengthens mucous membranes in the nose, mouth and throat, says Dr. Haas. Take one to two capsules twice a day at the onset of your symptoms. But don't take goldenseal on a regular basis because too much of it can irritate your liver, Dr. Haas cautions.

Toothache

• Sharp, recurring pain in one or more teeth

• Your tooth hurts when exposed to hot or cold, or when you eat sugar

What It ? Means

If you have pain in one or more teeth, read on. But once you've gotten relief, turn to page 33 and read how you could have avoided the problem in the first place. Chances are that you haven't been to the dentist for a long time and that you probably have a cavity.

Cavities are tooth holes that eventually get clogged with food. It's the getting-clogged part that sends the "Yeow!" signal to your brain.

Cavities aren't the only cause of tooth pain. Gnawing on hard pretzels or chewing on hard pizza crust can push your gums down, exposing parts of your tooth that have never before been open to air. Sudden changes in temperature—from drinking hot coffee while eating ice cream, for example—are going to make that tooth sting, says Dr. Charles H. Perle of the Academy of General Dentistry and the American Dental Association.

Symptom Solver

Let's say that, despite your best efforts—or because of your worst—you still wind up with a cavity or some other kind of tooth damage. There are no two ways about it: You have to see a dentist. But here are a few quick fixes that will help you feel better in the meantime.

Roll in the clove. To stop tooth pain fast, it often helps to clean out the cavity by rinsing or flossing or by using a toothpick. Then put a little oil of clove on a cotton ball and press it on the tooth. "That will provide temporary overnight relief until you get to the dentist's office," says Dr. Perle. Oil of clove is a nonprescription product available at drugstores and health food stores.

Pack it on ice. If the area around the tooth is swelling, apply an ice pack or frozen washcloth to the side of your face, being sure to either apply petroleum jelly on your skin or put the cold surface in a plastic bag in order to prevent burning your skin. Cold causes blood vessels to constrict, reducing swelling. Don't use heat, adds Dr. Perle. "Heat intensifies the nerve damage," he says. "It will drive you through the roof and cause increased swelling."

Forget the shortcut. Over-the-counter painkillers like aspirin or ibuprofen, taken orally, can help ease the pain. Don't think that you can make them work faster by rubbing them directly on the tooth or gum. It will cause a chemical burn, Dr. Perle says.

Preventing Toothaches

You know the drill: Brush, floss and see your dentist regularly. In addition, here are a two toothsavers that aren't so obvious.

Kiss your honey good-bye. You already know that sweets like honey and refined sugar can be bad for your teeth. Try chewing sugarless gum or eating some low-fat cheese, like Monterey Jack or Cheddar, after noshing on sugary snacks. This will stimulate your mouth's protective saliva production, helping to neutralize acids that lead to tooth decay, says Dominick DePaola, D.D.S., Ph.D., president and dean of Baylor College of Dentistry in Dallas. Spicy foods like chili also can be used to make your mouth water.

Use a straw. If you drink a lot of sugar-packed soda, sip it through a straw. Take small sips and swallow it on impact rather than swishing it around in your mouth. "Your teeth are not thirsty," Dr. Perle says. The idea is to keep that bacteria-producing sugar away from your teeth.

Vision Problems

- Your arms aren't long enough to read the newspaper

- You have trouble seeing at close range

What It ? Means

You don't see newborns wearing glasses. That's because nearly all of us have perfect eyesight when we're born. But as we grow up, our eyesight gets worse. And a lot of the damage results from the way we use our eyes, says Dr. James L. Cox of Bellflower, California.

Our eyes were designed to see distances beyond 10 to 15 feet. That was perfect for our ancestors, who used the farsighted feature when hunting. But the ability to see antelope across a grassy veld doesn't necessarily pay off in the computer age, when the "hunt" involves seeing things close up, like computer screens.

"The closer something is, the more you need to focus on it," says Dr. Robert Abel, Jr., of Thomas Jefferson University. That means that the eyes work harder.

More than a third of people between the ages of 17 and 24 have some sort of vision problem. By the time we reach our mid-sixties or seventies, just about all of us will have trouble seeing objects close up. Just for fun, hold the stock page of your newspaper's financial section about an arm's length away and slowly move it closer to your face. If you're 20 years old, you'll probably be able to see the numbers clearly at 6 to 7 inches. At age 30, the distance increases to about 10 inches. At 40, it's increased to 13 inches.

Symptom Solver

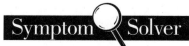

At some point in your life, you'll probably have to make a decision: Figure out a way to make your arms longer or see an eye doctor to get glasses or contact lenses. But there are a few ways to delay that day.

Strain to see. Like any other body part, the eyes benefit from exercise. Here's an easy workout: Try to read print that's slightly smaller than you are comfortable seeing, says Dr. Abel. Doing this periodically causes the eyes to work slightly harder, which will help keep them strong and flexible.

Here are some additional exercises that can help keep your eyes strong. Do one or more of these at least five times a day, says Dr. Cox.

- Move your eyes all the way to the right, all the way to the left and then up and down.
- Move your eyes in circles—clockwise and then counterclockwise.
- Hold your thumb at about the same distance you read at. Focus on it for a moment, then shift your gaze to a point across the room. Repeat several times, pausing at each place just long enough to get the object in focus.
- Hold your thumb in front of you an arm's reach away. Move it back and forth, up and down and in circles. Follow it with your eyes.

"Those movements make all of the systems of the eye work," says Dr. Cox. "You only have to do each exercise for 15 to 20 seconds, and you have the system all relaxed."

Set your sights on vegetables. Spinach and vegetables such as asparagus, red onions and garlic contain bioflavonoids and glutathiones, substances that are thought to slow down age-related vision loss, says Dr. Abel.

Vitamin A is another nutrient that's good for the eyes, says Dr. Abel. It's found in large amounts in foods such as carrots, pumpkin and sweet potatoes, he adds.

Take breaks. When working at a computer, take an eye break every 20 minutes. Look away from what you are doing and focus on something at least 15 feet away—across the room, down the hallway, out the window—to let your eyes rest, says Dr. Cox.

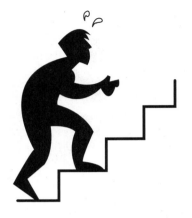

Part Three

Lungs and Heart

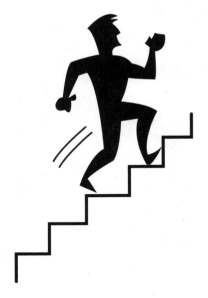

Breathing Problems

• You have shortness of breath at rest

• You develop breathlessness after exercise

• You are breathing rapidly

What It Means

If you're sucking wind after climbing a few flights of stairs, chances are good that you have health problems—but breathing may not one of them. (Trading your La-Z-Boy in the 'burbs for an exercise bike might not be a bad idea, however.)

But if you wake breathless at night, become breathless at rest, have a hacking cough day and night for a few months or start wheezing a few minutes into your morning jog, there's a chance that you've developed any one of several respiratory disorders that cause breathing problems.

"You can develop mild asthma, for example, and not know it until you exercise. But exercise isn't the cause. It's like cold air. Cold air doesn't cause it. It's a trigger," says Thomas Platts-Mills, M.D., Ph.D., director of the Division of Allergy and Clinical Immunology at the University of Virginia Medical Center in Charlottesville.

Like a well-planned subdivision, your respiratory system features a main entrance (your trachea) and is divided into two parts: the left and right main bronchi that supply air to your left and right lungs.

The goal of the whole operation is to take in air, break it down into various elements, keep the oxygen and send it to your bloodstream. The rest—nasty, harmful stuff like carbon dioxide, pollen and nicotine—is

removed or shunted back out of your body.

Normally, you're breathing easily—until some obstructive lung disease like asthma, bronchitis or emphysema moves in. Like bad neighbors with even worse friends, before long you have things like mucus building up along your once neatly groomed bronchi. Your bronchi are sometimes so appalled that they may even constrict—the very definition of an asthma attack touched off by pollen and dust allergens or cigarette smoke. And that wheezing you hear? Not Bob Dylan albums from next door, but narrowed airways resonating because of narrowing and excess mucus. Bronchitis features mucous secretion, inflammation and infection. Almost always caused by smoking, emphysema is the self-inflicted destruction of the lungs.

Ironically, some of the 13.1 million or more folks who suffer from asthma find that exercise—and sometimes only exercise—will trigger their attacks. What's worse is that the attack usually starts ten minutes into their workouts and peaks after the workouts stop. One possible reason: Your airways become cool and dry during exercise.

Allergies to a variety of plants like ragweed or pollen also can cause the airways to constrict or become congested with mucus. And some folks are so allergic to eggs, milk, soy, shrimp, peanuts or MSG (monosodium glutamate) that a single serving can leave them gasping.

Even your faithful pet Spike can cause breathing problems—although the evidence suggests that dogs are less likely to cause problems than cats. "The main environmental causes among children and young adults are clearly dust mites and house pets," says Dr. Platts-Mills.

Symptom Solver
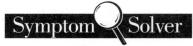

Since more than 5,000 people a year die from asthma, you don't want to fool around: See your doctor if you think you have asthma, says Dr. Platts-Mills. Keep a bronchodilator handy if you've already been diagnosed, he says. Meanwhile, consider these tips.

Protect yourself with a cup. For more than 100 years, coffee has been used by people to help with breathing problems like asthma, Dr. Platts-Mills says. "The caffeine molecule is very similar to that of the theophylline molecule—one of our treatments for asthma. For many patients, a cup of coffee will provide some relief," he says.

Munch on magnesium. Long known for its ability to relax the muscles lining our breathing passages, research shows that magnesium may even help fend off an asthma attack, says Richard J. Wood, Ph.D., associate professor at the School of Nutrition at Tufts University in Medford, Massachusetts, and Laboratory Chief of the Mineral Bioavailability Laboratory.

In a British study, researchers exposed more than 2,500 adults to a chemical that triggers airway constriction in asthma patients. As it turns out, those with the least magnesium in their diets were twice as likely to experience an asthmatic reaction as those with the highest magnesium diets. The Daily Value for magnesium is 400 milligrams, and some of the best sources are beans, nuts and dark green vegetables such as spinach and broccoli.

Lighten up. When suffering breathing problems like asthma, the last thing that you need is more pressure against the muscles that help control chest expansion and breathing. "Maintaining your ideal weight along with exercise can be helpful in controlling asthma," says Dr. Platts-Mills.

Do some redecorating. If you've been diagnosed with a sensitivity to a pet or dust mites, it's a good idea to get rid of an old sofa or carpets that serve as reservoirs for the allergens. "It's going to take three to four months to reduce cat allergen if you don't take pretty aggressive steps like getting rid of things," Dr. Platts-Mills says. If you can't part with the sofa or the carpets, steam clean them thoroughly, he says.

Launch a cover-up. To avoid further contamination by dust mites or dander, cover your mattresses and pillows with allergy-resistant materials, Dr. Platts-Mills says. He finds plastic covers or those obtained from an allergy-control company to be most effective. To receive more information on these, call Allergy Control Products at 1-800-422-3878.

Use a filter. Unfortunately, not just any department store model will do. "You probably should get an air-cleaning system with a high-efficiency particulate air (HEPA) filter. They're really the most effective," says Dr. Platts-Mills. It's basically a powerful air-filtering system that eliminates microscopic micron particles. Honeywell manufactures HEPA filtering systems called Enviracaire units. You can find out who sells them in your area by calling their toll-free number (1-800-332-1110). The prices range from $169 to $259.

Get in the swim of things. Swimming is one of the best exercises for people suffering from asthma because instead of inhaling dry air, which promotes cooling and water loss in the airways, you generally breathe warm, moist air when you swim, says Dr. Platts-Mills.

Ease into exercise. If you're committed to exercising on dry land, at least one study shows that you can prevent an asthma attack by taking 15 minutes to warm up. When 12 asthmatic people embarked on exercise without warming up, it only took six minutes before they had attacks.

But when the 12 participants did 15 minutes of moderate, continuous exercise before their run, half of them breathed with the ease of a nonasthmatic afterward. Walking, jogging and slow bicycling seem to be the best warm-up techniques, says Dr. Platts-Mills.

Head out early. Indoor exercise naturally cuts your exposure to air pollution and smog. But if you want to exercise outside, you may be better off exercising in the early morning in low-traffic areas, says Malcolm Blumenthal, M.D., director of the Section of Allergy at the University of Minnesota in Minneapolis. If you are allergic to certain pollens such as ragweed, however, you may want to head out later in the day when the counts may be lower.

Chest Pain

• You have discomfort, tightness or aching in the chest area

What It Means

It ranges in severity from mild discomfort to a pain so sharp and intense that it could have been delivered by the business end of a Louisville Slugger.

But when it comes to chest pain, we're with the experts: Don't take any chances. If you have any of the risk factors for heart disease—parents who have had heart attacks or you drink too much, smoke or are overweight—see your doctor. And soon. One out of six men are killed by heart disease—and you don't have to be one of them.

In fact, if you're just having chest discomfort, you should probably see a doctor, says Paul D. Thompson, M.D., director of preventive cardiology at the University of Pittsburgh Medical Center. "Men need to know that the first sign of heart problems is often not a pain, but discomfort. It can be a pain, but it doesn't have to be. And knowing that could save your life," says Dr. Thompson.

And remember this: Dangerous chest pain doesn't just radiate down your left arm, says Dr. Thompson. "You may feel it in your left arm, but it could just as easily be in your right arm, both arms, your neck and so on. I tell people that any discomfort from the earlobes all the way down to the belly button—especially if it comes on with exercise and goes away with rest—is something that you should talk over with your doctor promptly," says Dr. Thompson.

The Little Engine That Could

Why do you need to be concerned about chest pain or discomfort that only comes during strenuous activity? Think of your heart as the engine of your body, your arteries as fuel lines and your blood as the fuel. "When your engine is idling—your heart isn't beating hard—it doesn't need much fuel," says Dr. Thompson. Even clogged fuel lines—artery walls covered with fatty plaque—don't cause much trouble for an idling engine. But put the pedal to the metal—moving furniture, mountain biking, whatever—and those clogged fuel lines prevent your heart from getting the fuel that it needs to keep pumping, he says.

If you experience pain while moving, but it goes away after you catch your breath and rest for about 15 minutes, odds are that you have angina—the common name for clogged coronary arteries. More than three million men in the United States suffer from angina and the effects of coronary artery disease. Although patients often have trouble describing their pain, doctors say that there's a definite pattern. Most people come in with "discomfort, ache, much more on the dull end of the spectrum versus the sharper, there-is-a-pain-wow! kind of feeling," says L. Kent Smith, M.D., director of the preventive medicine programs at the Arizona Heart Institute in Phoenix.

Angina is the yellow caution flag on the Indianapolis Speedway of life. Ignore it, and you're headed for a crash—a heart attack. A heart attack occurs when fatty deposits or a blood clot block one of your arteries, completely cutting off the blood supply to a portion of your heart. The result is that part of your heart muscle can die.

The pain of a heart attack resembles angina but usually lasts longer, is more severe and may be accompanied by dizziness, nausea, shortness of breath and sweating. If you ever experience these symptoms, seek immediate emergency medical attention, says Dr. Smith.

Other potential causes of chest pain include inflammation of the pericardium, the small sac that contains your heart. This is usually caused by an upper respiratory infection. "You feel the most pain while you're lying down, and the pain lessens when you sit up and lean forward," says John D. Cantwell,

M.D., director of preventive medicine and cardiac rehabilitation at Georgia Baptist Medical Center in Atlanta and chief medical officer of the 1996 Olympic Games.

Also in the chest pain category is a heart muscle disorder called hypertrophic cardiomyopathy. "Often a patient will say that it feels like an elephant is sitting on his chest," Dr. Cantwell says. "This requires medical attention as well."

And of course, a five-alarm case of heartburn has been known to cause what feels like chest pain, but it's tough to tell the difference. "When in doubt, the best thing is to assume that it could be your heart and have it checked," says Jorge Herrera, M.D., associate professor of medicine at the University of South Alabama in Mobile. "People die from heart disease, but almost no one dies from heartburn or digestive problems."

Symptom Solver

If you're struck by pain or discomfort in the chest area, immediately inform your doctor or seek an emergency medical evaluation, says Dr. Smith. Here are some other steps that you can take to relieve the pain.

Stop. Immediately. Wherever you are, and whatever you're doing, sit down and rest, says Dr. Smith. If you are suffering from angina, the pain should go away in a few minutes. If it doesn't, or it gets worse, see your doctor—immediately. If the pain does go away, don't ignore this early warning sign. Discuss with your doctor the need for a medical evaluation.

Pop some antacid. While you're getting ready to visit your doctor, pop an antacid. If the pain goes away in a few minutes, it may have been heartburn after all—especially if you just ate, says Dr. Herrera.

Explore your family tree. One of the leading risk factors for heart disease is a relative who had a heart attack at a young age, says Dr. Cantwell. But if neither of your parents had a heart attack before age 70, your own chances of having one are much lower. "This would not apply if you are a smoker or have high

cholestrol levels," cautions Dr. Cantwell. "You have to look at the whole picture, health habits included, but if someone has a history of heart attack in his family and chest pain, there's good reason to be extra cautious. You'll want your doctor to monitor any chest pain no matter how minor you may think it is."

Heading Off a Heart Attack

Of course, the key is to avoid angina and other forms of heart disease. Here's how.

Take an aspirin every other day. In what may be one of the most interesting studies in medical history, 22,000 doctors between the ages of 40 and 80 were divided into two groups: those who were to take an aspirin every other day, and those who were to take a placebo or blank pill. Although the study was designed to run for five years, ethical considerations forced it to close well into its fourth. The reason is that a supervisory group discovered that fatal and nonfatal heart attack rates had been slashed in the aspirin group by 46 percent. "You can imagine the stir that that caused," Dr. Smith says. "Most people will benefit from this recommendation, and we know that it's safe."

Supplement with vitamin E. One study found that participants who took vitamin E for two years saw their risk of a nonfatal heart attack slashed by more than 70 percent, compared to a group that took placebos. However, Dr. Smith notes that this study only focused on people who already had narrowed coronary arteries. Still, observational studies tracking large groups of apparently healthy men and women showed a reduction in heart attacks by about one-third in those who took at least 200 International Units of vitamin E daily, says Dr. Smith.

Frolic with folic acid. Research suggests that if people would increase their daily total of folate to 400 micrograms, between 13,500 and 50,000 deaths from coronary artery disease could be prevented each year. That could reduce the risk of artery disease more than 10 percent for men. Folate, a B vitamin, is found in those dark green leafy vegetables that you may not have eaten since you last dined at your mom's house—broccoli, romaine lettuce and spinach.

The current Daily Value for folic acid—the supplement form of folate—is 400 micrograms. Since folic acid has been known to mask dangerous deficiencies in B_{12}, Shirley A. A. Beresford, Ph.D., study leader and epidemiologist at the University of Washington in Seattle, recommends that older men ask their doctors before taking supplements.

Get toasted. But not just any old toast will do. At least one study shows that eating bread made with flaxseed will help reduce cholesterol levels. During the study, 20 volunteers ate six slices of the bread a day for six weeks. At the end of the study, researchers found that LDL (low-density lipoprotein) cholesterol levels had dropped on average by 30 points.

"Wouldn't you rather take your medicine as a slice of toast with preserves or orange marmalade?" asks Tom Watkins, Ph.D., laboratory director of the Kenneth Jordan Heart Research Foundation in Montclair, New Jersey. "It sounds a lot better, doesn't it?"

A natural blood thinner, flaxseed apparently helps combat thickening of the blood that occurs as we age. Grind some up and sprinkle it over your cereal, says Dr. Watkins. You'll find flaxseed at your neighborhood health food store.

Give some blood. Most bloodmobiles provide a free cholesterol screening with each donation. And if your cholesterol level seems borderline high (between 200 and 239), then have yourself retested at a doctor's office, says Dr. Cantwell. If they exceed 240, see your doctor pronto.

Cut the fat. Research shows that eating less fat can reverse the amount of fat that builds up in your arteries. "You have to be careful not to overstate this, but when somebody has an artery that is 70 percent blocked and they go on a really low fat diet—maybe 10 percent fat—they might be able to bring that blockage down to 60 percent. They won't shrink it down to

normal, but it's definitely an improvement," says Dr. Smith.

Work it out. You don't have to beef up like Arnold Schwarzenegger. In fact, research suggests that moderate exercise may protect your heart just as well. "You don't need megadoses of exercise," says Dr. Smith. What you do need, he says, is "leisure-time physical activity of modest intensity." A brisk walk sustained for 20 minutes three or four times a week, for example, "begins to confer protection from a heart attack," says Dr. Smith.

Feed on fiber. In a six-year follow-up of the massive Health Professionals study, conducted at the Harvard School of Public Health, researchers found that men who ate more fruits, vegetables and especially cereals and grains were less likely to die from heart attacks. In fact, for every ten-gram increase in the amount of cereal fiber that the men ate, heart disease risk dropped by 29 percent, according to researchers.

Enjoy a fine wine. Research shows that a glass or two of wine a day does, indeed, help keep heart disease away. Doctors aren't sure why, but there is evidence that moderate alcohol consumption raises the level of good (HDL) cholesterol in the blood. So if you enjoy wine, by all means, continue to do so, says Dr. Smith. Just make sure that you limit yourself to one or two glasses. If you drink more on a regular basis, you start adding to your risk of high blood pressure and stroke, doctors warn.

Butt out for good. Research shows that cigarette smoking causes one-fifth of all heart disease deaths. Here's why. First, smoking makes it easier for cholesterol to enter the walls of your arteries, helping to accelerate atherosclerosis. Next, it can cause those same arteries to constrict. Finally, smoking causes platelets in your blood to get sticky.

The result? "You can take a narrowing of an artery that blood can barely get through and, with a little nicotine, block it off entirely and give yourself a heart attack," Dr. Thompson says.

Heartbeat Irregularities

- You feel your heart pounding at night
- You feel your heart racing during the day

What It Means

Imagine snapping your fingers 24 hours a day, seven days a week to a nonstop medley of show tunes. Though the verses often seem as if they've been specially designed for the rhythmically impaired, you're almost certain to miss a beat here and there.

Is it fair to expect better from your heart? Given that your heart beats about 100,000 times a day, an occasional irregular beat should almost be expected, says Dr. John D. Cantwell of Georgia Baptist Medical Center. "In a lot of cases, what the heart actually does is throw in a premature beat and then pauses until it gets back into its usual rhythm. With that many beats, you're asking a lot if you're expecting perfection."

In fact, one study shows that 43 percent of all adults experience at least one premature beat every 24 hours. The rest of us probably just don't notice. Of course, one form of irregular heartbeat, called arrhythmia, can be a sign of heart disease.

But if that's the case, you'll probably also experience chest pain and have a history of heart problems in your family. Fainting or an irregular heartbeat that keeps you up at night shouldn't be ignored either, says Dr. Cantwell. If you experience any of these symptoms, you should see a doctor, says Dr. Cantwell. (For more information on heart disease, see Chest Pain on page 64.)

What may seem like an abnormal heartbeat may actually be what's called a heart palpitation, often a fairly harmless—though annoying—problem.

"A palpitation is the sense that your heart is beating: You feel your heart beat, and you can feel your heart racing, your heart skipping, or pulsations in your neck," says Lou-Anne Beauregard, M.D., an electrophysiologist at Robert Wood Johnson University Hospital in New Brunswick, New Jersey.

"I wouldn't want to give anyone the impression that palpitations are totally benign, but on the other hand, I think that a lot of people who experience palpitations are having perfectly normal heartbeats," says Dr. Beauregard.

Since sorting out the difference is tricky stuff—and it is your ticker that we're talking about—it's probably a good idea to pay your doctor a visit whether you think you have palpitations or an arrhythmia.

"Your doctor might have you wear a monitoring device, which will allow him to determine the presence and specific nature of the heartbeat irregularities, some of which can be serious," says Dr. L. Kent Smith of the Arizona Heart Institute.

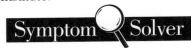
Symptom Solver

Take these tips into account as you consider your doctor's advice.

Mind your minerals. When it comes to keeping your heart's complex electrical system firing like a finely tuned engine, there are few minerals that are as important as potassium and magnesium. "If it's just a matter of an occasional skipped beat, and you've been reassured that it is not a potentially dangerous rhythm problem, you may find that it gets better if you supplement with these," says Dr. Beauregard.

The Daily Value for potassium is 3,500 milligrams. Have an eight-ounce glass of orange juice, a banana and a baked potato, and you're halfway there. The Daily Value for magnesium is 400 milligrams. An ounce of cashews and a three-ounce serving of halibut gives you almost half of what you need.

Be a moderate. An occasional drink shouldn't be a problem for most men. But getting tanked like you're some kind of aging fraternity rush chairman can cause not only heart arrhythmias but possibly a heart attack. "Although not everyone is susceptible to this condition, there's no other way to say it: Alcohol is poison to the heart," says Dr. Beauregard. "It precipitates abnormal rhythm by making the heart more irritable."

Go easy on the joe. Coffee bars are all the rage, but you may be better off ordering sparkling water if you're experiencing an irregular heartbeat, says Dr. Beauregard. Caffeine, a known stimulant, can cause your heart to race and, in some cases, skip beats, she says.

Hold the enchiladas. Some people reported fewer palpitations after they stopped eating jalapeño peppers and other spicy foods. "If you are ingesting something that seems to be correlated with increased symptoms, you should avoid it. I don't know why spicy foods seem to cause a problem, but patients tell me that they do," says Dr. Beauregard.

Trade sudden for steady. It's true: Some people are fast, and others are sudden. Those folks who shock their bodies with physical activity without taking the time to warm up in some way could be triggering their own arrhythmias. "Diving into cold water or suddenly running for a train after being a couch potato for the last five years can crank up your adrenaline and trigger abnormal rhythms," says Dr. Beauregard.

Do without certain decongestants. A small dose of decongestant may help relieve a stuffy nose, but too much is probably bad for your heart—especially products containing phenylpropanolamine and pseudoephedrine. Classified as stimulants, these chemicals seem to cause heart irregularities in folks who are strongly affected by caffeine. "These drugs are reasonably safe. You just need to make sure that you don't overdose on them," says Dr. Beauregard.

Chill with skill. Ever notice that your heart skips a beat when you eat something cold like ice or frozen yogurt? "It's probably because the esophagus is adjacent to one of the top chambers of the heart, and a sudden change in the temperature or a sudden slug of food going by can cause a little irritability," says Dr. Beauregard. Try eating frozen delights more slowly, but if it bothers you too much, consider seeing a doctor.

Take it off. "Although we look at each patient's overall health profile, being overweight could be a factor," says Dr. Cantwell. "The heart has to work harder to carry that extra weight around."

Say "time-out" to stress. For at least 30 minutes a day, bag the phone, beeper, fax machine or anything else that's keeping you on edge and hit the gym or the walking trail. "Once you've been properly diagnosed, I recommend stress reduction and exercise as ways of getting you to reduce and forget your palpitations," says Dr. Beauregard.

"You need to set aside 30 minutes as your inviolate time of day where you can do this and you won't be disturbed by anybody. Aerobic exercise not only strengthens the heart but releases beta endorphins in the brain that relieve stress—another heart-healthy benefit," she says.

Hang with a gang. What is a support group but a gang by another name, minus the tattoos? "The more serious the rhythm problem and stress in your life, the more I suggest that you get into a support group or counseling," says Dr. Beauregard. "In particular, I'm referring to guys in their forties, fifties and sixties who have had heart attacks in the past and continue to have abnormal heartbeats. Stress reduction can be a big help for these people."

Just say "no" to blow. Cocaine causes not only arrhythmias but heart attacks as well. "I see several of these a year," says Dr. Beauregard. "It's not pleasant."

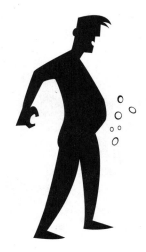

Part Four

Stomach and
Digestive System

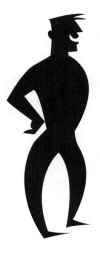

Anal Ailments

• Your anus is painful, itchy or bloody

What It ❓ Means

If you suffer from anal pain or bleeding, often constipation or even diarrhea are at the seat of your problem. "If the stool is very hard and dry, it essentially has to stretch the anus when it goes through. And that can cause a tear, called an anal fissure, or even a hemorrhoid as you strain," says Jorge Herrera, M.D., associate professor of medicine at the University of South Alabama in Mobile. (A hemorrhoid, by the way, is little more than a vein that has bulged out of your skin.)

Itching is another common symptom associated with hemorrhoids. In some cases it could mean pinworms—lowly creatures that normally infect children but can be spread to other members of the family. Or maybe some kind of fungus is homesteading in your rear.

Bleeding after a bowel movement is most commonly caused by those same angry inflamed hemorrhoids or an anal fissure, but bleeding also can be a symptom of a more serious problem. "Rectal bleeding can be a warning signal for colon cancer. But unless there is a family history of colon cancer at an early age, meaning younger than 50, colon cancer is not one of the most common causes. However, colon cancer should always be excluded because it's usually curable if detected at an early stage," says Dr. Herrera.

Symptom 🔍 Solver

Remember this rule of thumb: If you see blood, see a doctor.

If you're tired of being the butt of hemorrhoid jokes, here are some ways to help you sit comfortably again.

Chill out. Though not every expert agrees, you can find relief by either gently sitting on ice wrapped in a moist washcloth or wedging the ice-packed cloth in your upended booty. "It may sting at first, but it can be very helpful," says Colin Howden, M.D., professor of medicine at the University of South Carolina in Columbia. You may also want to try applying Tucks pads—an over-the-counter anal medication—that have been chilled.

Shed your workout gear. Since skin bacteria and fungus breed in warm, moist areas, shed your workout gear immediately after a trip to the gym, shower and slip into some cotton boxers or briefs, recommends Bruce Orkin, M.D., an assistant professor specializing in colon and rectal surgery at the George Washington University School of Medicine and Health Sciences in Washington, D.C. Both will help keep you dry and fungus-free.

Treat your butt better. Rather than torture yourself with that bargain-basement sandpaper you usually buy, spring for a softer bathroom tissue, maybe even one treated with soothing aloe vera. But be wary of those made with dyes or perfumes. They can cause itching and swelling, says David E. Beck, M.D., chairman of the Department of Colon and Rectal Surgery at Ochsner Clinic in New Orleans.

Fill up on fiber. Swear off that mushy, fat-and-sugar-laden junk food and get yourself a man-size serving of fiber every day. Eating unpeeled fruits and vegetables such as broccoli, cabbage, carrots and brussels sprouts will ward off constipation and diarrhea and, consequently, hemorrhoids and diarrhea, Dr. Herrera says.

Drink up. Wash that fiber down with six to eight eight-ounce glasses of water a day—more if you exercise or work in hot weather. Water also helps to keep you regular, Dr. Herrera says.

Slim down. If you started having problems with hemorrhoids at about the same time you had to buy new—and noticeably larger—pants, there may be a connection. Obesity has been known to cause hemorrhoids, says Dr. Herrera. So do your butt a favor and shed a few pounds.

Belching

- You're burping more than your Tupperware or your baby

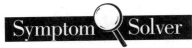
What It Means

Night after night, entertainer Don Ho knocks 'em dead with his signature song, "Tiny Bubbles." The popularity of the Hawaiian lounge legend and his ode to the intoxicating virtues of those little gaseous globules in his wine defies logic or explanation. Kind of like Wayne Newton and "Danke Schoen."

Now, it would be different if Ho belched in mid-song every time he mentioned those tiny bubbles. (Now, *that* we'd pay to see.) Because in real life, if you swallow enough of those tiny bubbles, they're going to find a way to come back up.

Trapped air is the fuel for that most masculine of pastimes: the fine art of belching. "Some people are compulsive air swallowers. They just blow themselves up like a balloon, and one of the only ways they can get it out is to burp it back up," says Malcolm Robinson, M.D., founder and director of the Oklahoma Foundation for Digestive Research and clinical professor of medicine at the University of Oklahoma College of Medicine in Oklahoma City.

Symptom Solver

We're not sure why anyone would want to stop, but here's how to squelch a belch—just in case.

Stop slurping. Drinking hot or cold liquids too fast or through a straw causes you to swallow air. Instead, drink slowly and lose the straw, says Dr. Robinson. You'll impress your pals with your newfound civility and belch less.

Slow down. Barking directives to your staff while gnawing on a sandwich not only makes you look like some Third World

potentate but also is another source of swallowed air. "You need to just slow down for a few minutes, take time to eat and then go back to what you're doing," says Dr. Colin Howden of the University of South Carolina.

Don't get chewed out. Okay, you've proven beyond any doubt that you can indeed walk and chew gum at the same time. But if you find yourself walking, chewing gum and belching at the same time, you might want to back up. Chewing gum can result in trapped air in your stomach and result in belching problems. And those problems are made worse when you're on the go. To top things off, if you're chewing sugarless gum, an ingredient called sorbitol not only will make you belch but also will give you gas, says Dr. Robinson (see Gas on page 74). We're not about to tell you to quit walking. That's good for you. But if you have a belching problem, you might want to try ditching the gum.

Pop the bubbles. There is no doubt that you already know that if you want to get into a belching contest with your buddies, the first thing you need is a beer, soda or some other carbonated beverage. But if you think that you're belching too much, can the carbonated drinks, advises Dr. Howden.

Send for the simethicone. Originally developed by the plastics industry to help remove air bubbles during manufacturing, simethicone is now an active ingredient in over-the-counter chewable tablets such as Gas-X and Mylanta Gas Relief. "Doctors even use it to clear bubbles out of your gastrointestinal tract while preparing for a procedure," Dr. Robinson says. "We put a little of this stuff in there, and then you have one big burp and all the little bubbles are gone."

Get heartburn help. Heartburn sufferers beware: In an effort to reduce the pain, you may be swallowing gallons of air a day. "If you notice this terrible bloated sensation, you're probably compensating for all that acid by swallowing too often and getting a stomach full of air," says Dr. Robinson. For ways to get relief, see Heartburn on page 75.

Constipation

- You haven't had a bowel movement in days

What It ? Means

As far as locker-room bull sessions go, it's a rare day—and thankfully so—that constipation is the topic of discussion. But the reason probably has less to do with the limits of polite conversation than the simple fact that active guys generally don't get constipated.

Among other things, exercise increases what's called bowel motility: literally, the speed at which your bowels move stuff through your colon. "Constipation is usually a combination of three things: lack of fiber, not enough exercise and not drinking enough fluids," says Dr. Jorge Herrera of the University of South Alabama.

In fact, exercise has such a big impact on bowel motility that some distance runners suffer from what's called runner's trots—diarrhea—obviously the opposite problem.

If you occasionally suffer from constipation, you're not grunting alone. It's the most common digestive complaint among U.S. males. And about 7 percent say that it's a chronic problem. There's no set quota of how many bowel movements a week are considered regular, although some doctors say that you generally should have at least three stools a week. But that figure varies widely, and the real key is whether there has been a sudden change in your habits lately.

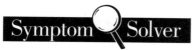

Symptom Solver

Try these tips to keep things moving smoothly.

Fiber up. Eating 20 to 30 grams of fiber a day is a good way to help you avoid constipation. "Probably the easiest way to get that in the diet is to eat salads and fresh fruits like apples and pears with the peels on. Also, choose breads with fiber, like wheat or oat bran," Dr. Herrera advises. (And no cutting off the crusts like Mom used to do for you when you lived at home). Some foods with the highest fiber contents are broccoli, cabbage, carrots and brussels sprouts—all the stuff you never eat.

Water yourself. It seems like enough liquid to float the U.S.S. Eisenhower, but you need to drink six to eight glasses (eight ounces each) of water a day to keep your stool soft and avoid constipation, says William B. Ruderman, M.D., attending physician for Gastroenterology Associates of Central Florida in Clearwater. And if you're eating all the fiber that you're supposed to, you may need even more.

Do without dairy. An insoluble protein found in milk and cheese called casein has been found to plug up the bowels of some. Eating low-fat foods also helps you stay a regular guy.

Name the first Moody Blues hit. Stumped? Time's up. It was "Go Now." And that's precisely what you should do if your body tells you that it's time to go to the bathroom. If you delay too long, the gut reabsorbs water from the stool that's trying to find a way out. And that turns the stool from soft to hard. Now, consider the opening through which all things must pass and then decide: Would you rather have a scoop of mashed potatoes or a golf ball trying to squeeze through?

Check your medicine cabinet. Prescription antidepressants and painkillers, as well as over-the-counter antacids containing aluminum, have all been found to cause constipation, says Dr. Colin Howden of the University of South Carolina.

Stir up some fiber. Over-the-counter fiber products such as Metamucil and Citrucel are designed to be added to juice or water, says Dr. Howden. Also added to water or juice, psyllium is a natural-fiber laxative that aids constipation. Psyllium is available in most health food stores and some grocery stores.

Diarrhea

• You have a sudden need to go to the bathroom, followed by loose stools

What It Means

Many a road racer has been chugging toward the finish line only to discover that he has to make a pit stop behind the nearest tree.

"We don't know for sure why this happens, but we think that running decreases the transit time of food in the intestine—things just move through faster," says Gary Green, M.D., associate team physician of intercollegiate athletics at the University of California, Los Angeles.

More common are the bacterial causes of diarrhea. Shaking hands with someone who hasn't washed theirs, eating from the same buffet table, using the same glass—all can quickly spread the kind of microscopic bugs that wreak havoc on your digestive system. "One of two things happens: The bacteria either attack the absorbing mechanisms in your small intestine or speed intestinal motility," says Arnold Wald, M.D., professor of medicine at the University of Pittsburgh Medical Center.

Although such gastrointestinal distress is less than charming, it's usually not harmful and lasts, at most, a week. Bloody diarrhea or diarrhea accompanied by fever are obviously more severe and can be symptoms of what's called dysentery, Dr. Wald warns. If you think that that's what you have, consult your doctor.

Symptom Solver

If your stomach has you on the runs, here are some ideas sure to bring fast relief.

Be clear. "A clear liquid diet of things like Jell-O, apple juice and soft drinks will sometimes stop diarrhea cold," says Dr. Malcolm Robinson of the Oklahoma Foundation for Digestive Research. "If you eat food, you will get more diarrhea. It's that simple."

Bye, milk. Lactose intolerance—the inability to digest the sugar in milk—is a common cause of diarrhea. "Even if you drink milk without difficulty today, you could lose your ability to tolerate it as you get older," Dr. Robinson cautions.

Go for a bland-aid. If you have to eat, stick with foods like bananas, rice and toast and avoid fat at all costs. "Eating bananas is particularly good because it helps replenish potassium that is lost when you have diarrhea," says Dr. Wald.

Skip the caffeine. You may want to cut caffeine out of your diet until your digestive woes pass. "It seems to stimulate the speed at which your bowels work—especially if you exercise," Dr. Green says. Caffeine, like alcohol, is a diuretic, which makes the fluid loss associated with diarrhea that much worse.

Eat and run—but carefully. If you have problems with runner's trots, stick with carbohydrate and electrolyte solutions like Gatorade. Low-fat and fiber energy bars work, too, says Dr. William B. Ruderman of Gastroenterology Associates of Central Florida. Just make sure that you eat at least an hour before you hit the track. In fact, high-fiber meals containing whole grains, dried fruits and nuts and seeds are to be avoided even the day before a race.

Chew on this one. Does your sugarless chewing gum contain sorbitol? It could be causing your diarrhea, says Dr. Robinson. When bacteria in your colon sink their teeth into sorbitol, they break it down, creating lots of gas and causing water to flow into your stools. The result is pain and diarrhea.

Keep your eye on antacids. Antacids made with magnesium are helpful for heartburn, but they have the nasty habit of pulling water into your intestine—a prime cause of diarrhea. If you need to take antacids, try using less, or alternate with one made with calcium, Dr. Robinson advises.

Gas

- They call you Mr. Methane

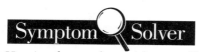

What is it about farting that at once fascinates and disgusts us? If we release one of our own, we think to ourselves, hey, that's not so bad. In fact, it smells kind of . . . interesting, like musk, perhaps. But let someone else light one up, and we're among the first to announce: "Buddy, something must have crawled up in you and died!"

Not that you're worried about his health or anything, but even the most malodorous flatulence rarely signals a problem. Gas is merely the end result of good bacteria in your intestine helping break down your food. Difficult-to-digest foods like beans, for example, produce the most gas, but no matter what you eat, studies show that, on average, we break wind a minimum of 14 times a day.

Anyway you cut it, that's a lot of "musk."

Symptom Solver

Here's what to do to rid yourself of gas.

Banish the milk cow blues. Remember that government-funded study a few years back? The one where they were trying to figure out if cows were poking holes in the ozone layer by passing too much gas? They would have been better off looking into what happens when humans digest products that come from those cows.

After you drink milk or eat milk-based products, an enzyme in your duodenum called lactase is supposed to digest a sugar in the milk called lactose. The problem is that some people are what doctors call lactase-deficient, meaning that they no longer have the enzyme. The result is lots of gas. If you're one of those, fear not.

"You could either take the lactase tablets or capsules, which are available over the counter, or drink milk that has the lactose removed, like Dairy Ease or Lactaid," says Dr. Malcolm Robinson of the Oklahoma Foundation for Digestive Research.

Scratch sorbitol. Not only will chewing gum make you swallow air—a common cause of gas—but sugarless brands are often made with an ingredient known as sorbitol, says Dr. Robinson. "This stuff is famous for getting into your colon and making lots of gas," he says. Diet candies and other diet products also frequently contain sorbitol. So if you think that you're passing wind too much, pass on the sorbitol.

Find a new fiber supplement. If you've noticed more gas since you began using a fiber supplement, consider switching to another brand. "That seems to be enough to do the trick for some people," says Dr. Jorge Herrera of the University of South Alabama.

Buy some Beano. If you like to eat beans, you might want to invest in Beano, an over-the-counter product that helps your body break down beans before methane and hydrogen are created. "Some people say that Beano is the greatest thing in the world; others say it's worthless. . . . I guess it depends on why you have gas. If you are a person who has gas because you are eating too many beans or things like cauliflower or broccoli, it should work," says Dr. Robinson.

Cut back on protein products. High-fiber vegetarian fare may make you pass gas more, but eating lots of protein in the form of meat and eggs may make your gas smell worse. It's the old quantity-versus-quality debate. "There's a wonderful book that was written in Japan for kids called *The Gas We Pass*. It explains that carnivores, meat-eaters, like lions, have bad-smelling gas, but animals like cows or horses who are vegetarians make a lot of gas that doesn't smell so bad. So if you want to have nice-smelling gas, I guess you should be a vegetarian," Dr. Robinson says.

Heartburn

• You have a painful burning sensation in your stomach and, sometimes, your chest

What It Means

You start the day with a large cup of coffee and a smoke. Then you inhale a giant Italian sub with onions and hot peppers for lunch. For dinner, you scarf down a huge plate of Buffalo chicken wings—washed down, naturally, by several pitchers of beer. And as you lie down at night, you get heartburn so bad that it brings tears to your eyes.

Of course, you know why. It was that spicy chicken wing sauce, on top of those onions and peppers that you had for lunch. Right?

Wrong.

"It's not the spice that gets you; it's the fat and the smoke and the alcohol," says Dr. Jorge Herrera of the University of South Alabama. "Many of these guys are overweight, too. All four things combine to give you a terrible case of heartburn."

If you're having heartburn and still smoking and eating and drinking too much, you need to—first and foremost—move out of the frat house. *National Lampoon's Animal House* was a comedy—not a lifestyle documentary. Besides, a man your age should at least have his own apartment. And you should probably see a doctor as well. There's a possibility that you're actually suffering from cardiovascular disease or having a mild heart attack.

"The pain can be similar. When in doubt, the best thing is to assume that it's the heart and have it checked," says Dr. Herrera. If you have a family history of heart problems, though, see a doctor anyway—you need to talk with him about your diet. For more information about heart problems, see Chest Pain on page 64.

As for you heartburn sufferers, ever wonder why it hurts so much? In a healthy gastrointestinal tract, acid stays in the stomach, helping to break down food. The only thing separating this powerful acid and your esophagus is a small muscle that squeezes open and closed, called your lower esophageal sphincter.

Weaken that small muscle any number of ways—eating too much fat, drinking too much booze or smoking cigarettes, for example—and stomach acid is free to lap at your tender esophagus, causing pain.

"All you need is a little bit of acid in there to cause problems, because the esophagus is not used to handling it," says Dr. Gary Green of the University of California, Los Angeles.

And athletes who overindulge in the wrong stuff and then exercise are prime candidates for big-time heartburn, Dr. Green says.

Symptom Solver

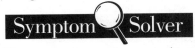

There are plenty of ways to beat the burn. Try these.

Chew gum. Saliva generated by gum chewing can help put out the fire in your esophagus, Dr. Herrera says.

Lose your love handles. Carrying just 15 percent more weight on your frame increases your likelihood of heartburn. Some studies have shown that excessive weight can reduce the holding power of the esophageal sphincter. Those extra pounds also increase the upward pressure of stomach acids. (And until you lose the weight, lose those tight clothes, says Dr. Herrera. They can cause stomach pressure, too.)

Tilt that bed. If you have chronic heartburn, you can ease your nighttime bouts and simultaneously create a low-rent version of an adjustable bed. Simply place the two legs at the head of the bed on bricks or blocks of wood. The angle will help prevent acid from seeping from your stomach into your esophagus while you sleep, says Dr. Green.

Think before you drink. Although mugs of coffee and alcohol may top your list of favorite beverages, you can help reduce your heartburn by drinking less of both. Coffee and alcohol not only decrease the strength of the esophageal muscle but also increase stomach acid production, says Dr. William B. Ruderman of Gastroenterology Associates of Central Florida.

And even switching to decaf might not help. "There are studies that show that it's not so much the caffeine as the oils in the coffee," adds Dr. Herrera. Red wine also has a reputation for causing heartburn.

Launch a pre-emptive strike. Heart set on a night of pizza and beer with the boys but worried about a major-league case of heartburn? Drop some antacid one hour before the big feast and three hours after, says Dr. Herrera. "That way, you'll blunt the acid throughout the period when it's being produced," he says. "That's the good thing about antacids. They work almost immediately. If you know that certain foods are going to cause heartburn, you can prevent it by taking an antacid before."

Trim that fat. Eating less fat can save you from heartburn. "Fatty foods delay the emptying of the stomach, so you can just imagine how that would put pressure on the esophageal muscle," says Dr. Green. Some of the worst offenders are fried foods and chocolate, he says.

Drink milk. Although not all doctors agree, some suggest that in a pinch, a glass of milk might help your heartburn. "Compared to what you can buy at the store, milk is a fairly weak antacid. But it can improve symptoms for a short time," says Dr. Herrera.

Pass on the peppermint. Ever wonder why you seem to develop heartburn after visiting a restaurant that serves peppermints with the bill? It's probably not the size of the check—although that could be a

The Tooth Decay Connection

It's bad enough that you feel like the whale in *Pinocchio*, when that annoying little insect Jiminy Cricket and his wooden-headed friend lit a fire in its belly. Now it turns out that your bouts with heartburn may be slowly eating away at your teeth.

A University of Alabama, Birmingham, study of 30 patients with chronic heartburn found that more than two-thirds of them also showed some degree of dental erosion. It seems that when digestive acids from the stomach sneak past your lower esophageal sphincter, they can creep up into the throat and mouth. Tooth enamel that is subject to frequent contact with the refluxed stomach acid can develop its own type of "heartburn"—it begins to erode.

"This is not to say that everyone who gets heartburn is doomed to have eroded teeth," says Patrick Schroeder, M.D., gastroenterologist, formerly with the University of Alabama, now at Good Samaritan Hospital in Kearney, Nebraska. "But since dental erosion is difficult to spot in its early stages, it can't hurt to minimize any risk you may have by talking to your doctor or dentist."

factor. Peppermint also weakens the esophageal sphincter, says Dr. Herrera.

Eat right before you exercise. Olympic records have certainly been set on some pretty weird precompetition diets, but if you have problems with heartburn, stick with carbohydrate and electrolyte solutions like Gatorade no sooner than an hour before you work out, Dr. Green says.

Mind your medication. Aspirin, anti-inflammatory pills and certain heart, blood pressure and asthma medications can all increase stomach acid production, Dr. Herrera says.

Incontinence

- You're dribbling more than the Harlem Globetrotters

- You wet yourself when you sneeze or laugh

- You know that you have to go, but you can't hold it for the short time that it takes to get to the bathroom

What It ? Means

Nobody ever accused you of being a plumber, but if your kitchen faucet dripped for a couple of weeks, you'd eventually pull out the channel locks and have at it. One on one. Just you against the pipes.

Same thing with incontinence, or the accidental leakage of urine. Whether it's just a few drops or an embarrassing deluge, "urinary leakage is never normal and needs treatment," says Cindy Maloney, a family nurse practitioner and director of the Incontinence Treatment Center in Troy, New York. "It's always a symptom of an underlying problem. But once that's diagnosed, it's just a matter of taking advantage of the different treatment options."

Few guys have problems with incontinence until they reach their fifties. On the other hand, roughly one in four women between age 39 and 59 suffers from this liquid injustice. Why? Not only is a woman's bladder smaller, but her plumbing gets worked over while she's pregnant. Suffice it to say, there's a lot of jostling and stretching going on during those nine months.

A healthy male bladder has no such problem. Sitting unmolested behind the pelvis, it expands like a water balloon as urine pours in from the kidneys. Once full, you get the high sign that it's time to excuse yourself and make your way to the bathroom—no runs, drips or

errors. Standing in front of a urinal, you absent-mindedly relax the urinary sphincter (a ringlike muscle that holds urine in), allowing urine to drain through the urethral canal, past the prostate and out of the penis. Your only real concern is making sure that you zip your fly.

Not so if you're suffering from one of the many forms of incontinence. If, for example, you're dribbling small amounts of urine all day, that's called overflow incontinence. Experts say that it's possible that your prostate is swollen and has begun to prevent your bladder from emptying, causing it to spill. "Think of your bladder as a barrel that you fill with fluid—and you keep filling it until it overflows. That's overflow incontinence," says L. Dean Knoll, M.D., director of research at the Center for Urological Treatment and Research in Nashville.

The good news is that although swelling of the prostate is as inevitable as gray hair—more than half of the male population over age 50 and three-quarters over age 70 have an enlarged prostate—it only causes overflow incontinence in a small percentage of men, according to Dr. Knoll.

Men who have had their prostates removed or operated on—usually because of cancer or excessive swelling—more commonly suffer from what's called stress incontinence. Simply sneeze, laugh or lift something at the wrong time and you're liable to get wet.

If your bladder tells your brain to find a bathroom right away, only to empty en route, that's urge incontinence—another potential calling card of an enlarged prostate.

And then there's that uniquely male habit of waiting until the last possible second to go. This can do more than make you damp when you miscalculate. Over time, it can stretch your bladder, which may contribute to incontinence down the road.

Weak urinary sphincter muscles can also be a source of persistent dribbling, although this is much more common in women because of childbearing and menopause. In addition, Alzheimer's disease, diabetes, infections, multiple sclerosis, prescription drugs and constipation have all been linked to incontinence.

What *isn't* incontinence is the little bit you occasionally spill on your khakis when you forget to give a good shake. That's not a health problem, man. You're just moving too fast.

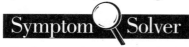

Whether you have a slow leak or a flood, here's how to dam the flow.

Show your bladder who's boss. When nature calls, do you come running? Maybe it's time to put yourself in charge. Try drinking a little less fluid so that you only have to go to the bathroom every three to four hours. This will help keep your bladder under your command so that it only goes when you're ready—and not before. "It's a very reasonable approach that can have good results," says Dr. Knoll.

Be careful with medicines. A number of over-the-counter products, such as insomnia medications, cough suppressants and antihistamines, cause the bladder to retain urine. If your prostate is already swollen, it could press on the bladder, causing overflow incontinence. "Someone with just a mildly swollen prostate could develop incontinence," Maloney says.

Consider taking Sudafed. "This medication causes constriction under the bladder neck; it can definitely help with stress incontinence," says Maloney. Most doctors, however, don't recommend using it for long periods of time, or if a person has specific health problems, like hypertension. "You need to go to a doctor to make sure that you're not causing additional problems with your bladder," she adds.

Be picky with prescriptions. Some wonder drugs work wonders; others can cause you to spring a leak. Drugs such as beta-blockers, diuretics, antidepressants and sleeping pills have all been known to cause incontinence.

Check with your doctor if you suspect that your medications are causing problems.

Think before you drink. You don't have to swear off coffee and an occasional beer, but be aware that alcohol and caffeine irritate the lining of the bladder—which can make you urinate more often, says Maloney. Other potential bladder irritants include artificial sweeteners, fruit juices, spicy foods and even milk. "The bottom line is that if someone is having incontinence and he drank a lot of these, it could aggravate his problem."

Unblock those bowels. Constipation is bad for many reasons, but here's one more: It puts pressure on the bladder, which can lead to incontinence, says Maloney. The best way to relieve constipation is to eat more dietary fiber in the form of whole grains, fruits and vegetables (see Constipation on page 72).

Strengthen that sphincter. You'll never see them displayed in bodybuilding competitions (we hope), but strong sphincter muscles are mighty important, particularly in men who have had prostate surgery, Dr. Knoll says.

Before you can strengthen the urinary sphincter, you have to find it. The next time you're urinating, stop the flow for a moment. (We'll wait here while you do it.) The muscle that stops the flow is the urinary sphincter. To make this muscle stronger, experts recommend squeezing it 50 times in a row, at least three times a day. You can do this at your desk or even while standing in line at the bank. "For some, it will help control leaking," says Dr. Knoll.

Consider collagen. If your urologist finds that your urinary sphincter lacks the bulk to close properly, he may recommend a strategically placed collagen injection to fill the gap, says Dr. Knoll.

Get to know your doctor. Since swelling of the prostate gland is a common cause of incontinence in men, it's probably a good idea to get the little doodad checked. In fact, you should pay your primary care doctor a visit every year after age 40, says Maloney.

Nausea/Vomiting

• Your stomach is irritated, queasy or upset

• You feel like you're in a hurling contest—and we're not talking about the Irish sport

What It ? Means

When former President George Bush vomited on the Japanese prime minister during a dinner held in that country, some viewed it as the barf hurled round the world.

In fact, it was probably a defensive act by the former president. Not against Japanese cuisine, but against microscopic viruses that had invaded his gut and, once detected by his brain's vomit control center, needed to be expelled. Think of it as your body's own version of the ejector seat in James Bond's car. If there's a villain sitting there, pointing a gun at our hero, the bad guy's going to be thrown up—and away.

It's unlikely that your nausea or vomiting will ever become an international incident, leading network newscasts, fueling comedians' jokes for weeks and sparking reams of magazine and newspaper coverage. (Unless, of course, *you* barf on a president—a practice, by the way, not generally well-received by the Secret Service.) But the cause may be the same: gastric flu inadvertently passed along in a buffet line or through some other form of casual contact. Though gastric flu is tough to self-diagnose, you'll probably have additional symptoms like a fever or chills.

There's far less mystery about alcohol-induced nausea: You've gone to the well one too many times, and as a matter of survival, your body is kicking it back up.

Nausea that occurs once after a meal often means that Aunt Mildred's potato salad wasn't quite as fresh as she had advertised and is riddled with bacteria. Regardless of the cause, however, all have nearly the same result.

"Nausea is a protective mechanism. If there's something in there that shouldn't be, it's ejected from your body," says Dr. Colin Howden of the University of South Carolina.

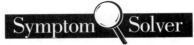
Symptom Solver

Rather than fight the feeling, sometimes it's just better to let yourself vomit. If you can't or haven't, try these tips to soothe your stomach.

Ask for the real thing. Defizzed Coke works so well for nausea that there's an over-the-counter product on the market called Emetrol that is made of essentially the same thing. "It's basically a high-fructose, sweet, syrupy medicine that is just like Coke syrup. I'm not sure how it works, but it must get the job done, because it's something that people have been using for years," says Dr. Malcolm Robinson of the Oklahoma Foundation for Digestive Research. You can make your own by simply opening a Coke and stirring it for a few minutes until it's flat.

Make like Gilligan. Like everyone else on *Gilligan's Island*, he was always trying to get his hands on Ginger. (Of course, we always preferred Mary Ann.) Some studies show that the herb ginger works nearly twice as long as the anti-motion sickness drug Dramamine—without the side effects. You can drink ginger tea, or—for more intense nausea—try ginger capsules of 400 milligrams, available in many health food stores, suggests researcher Daniel Mowrey, Ph.D., director of the American Phytotherapy Research Laboratory in Salt Lake City. Follow label instructions for dosage. If you don't have any ginger on hand, drink ginger ale.

Eat light. If you feel nauseated, eat only low-fat, plain foods, such as saltines, says

Robert M. Stern, Ph.D., a researcher on motion sickness and nausea for NASA and professor of psychology at Pennsylvania State University in University Park. High-fat foods take hours to digest, while lighter foods can ease stomach pain and are easily digested.

If you're vomiting, Dr. Stern says, don't eat anything for at least one hour, since it will take your stomach that long to settle. Then, he suggests, have small portions of bread, broth or other bland foods.

Go easy with pain relievers. Taking ibuprofen or aspirin for a few days isn't a problem. But extended use—ten days or more—increases your risk for another possible cause of nausea: gastric ulcer, warns Dr. Jorge Herrera of the University of South Alabama. "At the same time that you're trying to reduce your pain, you're weakening the defense of your stomach, and these pain relievers can start digging a hole in there," he says. On the other hand, over-the-counter products containing acetaminophen do not cause ulcers.

Break out the Pepto-Bismol. Nauseated from drinking too much? Take some Pepto-Bismol. "Nobody knows all the things that Pepto-Bismol does, but for people who have nausea as a result of some kind of irritation of the stomach, Pepto-Bismol is very effective," Dr. Robinson says. Just be aware that using it for a few days can turn stools dark.

Get checked for an ulcer. If your nausea persists and doesn't seem to be associated with drinking too much, ask your doctor to test you for an ulcer, says Dr. Herrera.

The Motion, the Ocean and You

Deep inside your brain is the name of the first girl you ever made out with and something called your chemoreceptor trigger zone—also known as your vomit control center. Hopefully, the two aren't located in close proximity.

The rocking of a ship is almost guaranteed to send off alarms in your vomit control center. The problem is that while your eyes may be fixed on a lounge chair or cabana, the fluid inside your inner ear continues to rock, giving your vomit control center the high sign to let it fly. To avoid embarrassment, try these tips.

Watch the horizon. Instead of staring at a single object within the rocking scene, you should look immediately at the horizon. This should tame your nausea in no time, says Dr. Malcolm Robinson of the Oklahoma Foundation for Digestive Research.

Press away nausea. The Chinese technique of acupressure can short-circuit motion sickness, says Kenneth Koch, M.D., professor of medicine at the Milton S. Hershey Medical Center at Pennsylvania State University in Hershey. The acupressure spot is located exactly in the middle of your wrist, three finger widths down from the wrinkle that separates your palm and your wrist. You can buy elastic acupressure wristbands that exert constant pressure on the correct point at many sporting goods stores. "I'm not sure if they work or not, but I've had patients tell me that they love them," says Dr. Robinson.

Buy some relief. "Dramamine and Benadryl are extremely closely related: They are medicines that work on the nausea center. They aren't always effective, but they aren't dangerous either," Dr. Robinson says.

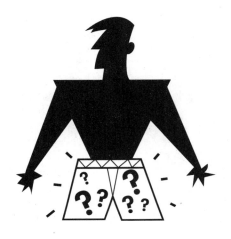

Part Five

Sexual Organs

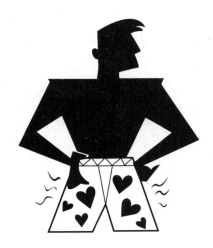

Impotence

- You're not able to get an erection 20 percent of the time

- You can't maintain an erection

- You're performing intercourse that's not satisfying to you or your partner at least 20 percent of the time

What It Means

Imagine that you're a Little League baseball coach, and you have a big kid—let's call him Woody—batting cleanup. Now Woody's been known to really stroke the ball, but tonight, with bases loaded, inexplicably, he fans. Do you bench him for the rest of the season? Or in calm tones reassure the young lad that tomorrow is another day?

Any would-be Lou Pinella knows that an encouraging word is usually enough to put Woody back on track. Another couple of bad nights, and it would be wise to make sure that his fundamentals are still sound—that he hasn't slipped into any bad habits, for example. A dramatic drop in his batting average may signal a more severe problem.

So it is with that *other* national pastime. If your sex life has become a series of scoreless innings because of impotence, don't panic. There are several reasons why you might not be able to get an erection, but there's a good chance that specific lifestyle changes and medical treatment can help you overcome your slump.

Perhaps foremost to remember: You're not alone. An estimated 10 to 15 million men have varying degrees of the same problem. Untold others—when stressed and harried and their minds are elsewhere—occasionally can't get it up. "I mean, my gosh, everybody strikes out once in a while," says Sheldon Burman, M.D., founder and director of The Male Sexual

Dysfunction Institute in Chicago.

So keep in mind that even such prodigious Hall of Fame sluggers as Babe Ruth, Mickey Mantle and Reggie Jackson struck out a lot. In fact, Jackson—whose home run heroics earned him the nickname "Mr. October"—fanned once in every four at bats. That may be acceptable for major league power hitters, but in the bedroom, you want to make contact almost every time. If, however, you can't get an erection about one time in five, your penis may actually be trying to alert you to some potentially serious health problems. "Cigarette smoking, diabetes, cardiovascular disease, coronary artery disease, hypertension—we now know that they're all causes of impotence," says L. Dean Knoll, M.D., director of research at the Center for Urological Treatment and Research in Nashville.

Consider the effect of cardiovascular disease on a healthy penis. When you're sexually aroused, biochemicals like prostaglandin E_1 relax the arteries leading to your penis, allowing blood to flow more freely down there.

Also relaxed by the effects of prostaglandin, the spongy, cavernous tissue that makes up the body of your penis quickly fills with all that onrushing blood. Of course, owning an engorged penis is nice, but it still isn't quite enough. The veins and tissue then have to constrict at just the right time to keep the blood in place—another function of prostaglandin. If all goes well, you have an erection that should last until orgasm. The process is so natural; it's one of those things that you really can do in your sleep. In fact, most men get two to four erections a night while they're off in dreamland.

Over time, bad eating habits and lack of exercise can cause waxy plaque to build up inside the blood vessels of the penis. "The arterial walls narrow, and so the velocity or the amount of blood that can move through this artery is decreased. As the amount of blood is decreased, you don't fill the spaces in the body of the penis needed to obtain and maintain good-quality erections," says Dr. Knoll. And because blood vessels leading to the penis are less than half the size of those carrying blood to the heart, impotence can be a tip-off that you might be on your way to heart disease, he says.

In fact, nearly anything that harms your vascular health can contribute to impotence. If you're able to get an erection—only to have it wilt within a few minutes—experts say that you may be suffering from leaky veins. Unable to clamp down properly, these tiny varicose veins allow the blood to pour back into circulation—leaving you limp, says Dr. Burman.

Fifty to 60 percent of all men with diabetes will experience impotency. "If I see 20 patients today, probably 5 or 6 of them are going to be suffering from diabetes," says Dr. Burman. Often a symptom of the nerve and vascular damage related to diabetes, impotence may appear without warning. "As best as we can tell, they get hardening of the arteries a little sooner and a little more severely than folks who aren't diabetic. And they don't have the smooth synchronized interaction that they need between nerves," he says.

Most experts agree that medications taken for other illnesses may cause a quarter of all impotence cases. Among them are anti-anxiety drugs and antidepressants like fluoxetine hydrochloride (Prozac); prostate treatments like tetrazosin hydrochloride (Hytrin), doxazosin mesylate (Cardura), and finasteride (Proscar); arthritis and ulcer medications like cimetidine (Tagamet) and ranitidiine hydrochloride (Zantac); a few blood pressure drugs and some painkillers. (You should never discontinue the use of any prescription drugs without consulting your doctor.) Persistent use of addictive substances

The Flip Side

To those suffering from impotence, it sounds like the dream disease: an erection that lasts for hours. But there's a price to be paid for that stubborn stiffy, called priapism by the guys in white lab coats. Left untreated for several hours, priapism can cause pain and permanent damage to your penis.

"You can develop scar tissue in the penis, which will not allow your erection to work well from then on," says John Mulcahy, M.D., professor of urology at Indiana University Medical Center in Indianapolis.

At one time, the most common causes of priapism were penile injuries, some spinal diseases and sickle cell disease. But doctors say that the problem has, well, been on a slight rise since phentolamine mesylate (Regitine) and that prostaglandin E_1 injections have become a medical treatment for impotence. While most men don't have any side effects, a few will develop priapism after this kind of treatment, says Dr. Mulcahy.

So what's to be done with an endless erection? A shot of epinephrine or phenylephrine causes blood vessels to shrink, which is usually enough to bring it back down to resting size, he says.

such as alcohol, marijuana and cocaine also are known to cause impotence in many cases.

Like the confident trot of a home run hitter, your ability to get an erection also slows as the seasons of life pass. "As men get older, it takes longer to get aroused. It takes more stimulus to get a good-quality erection. It also may mean that it takes longer to get an erection after having an orgasm," says Dr. Knoll. In fact, roughly one man in three over the age of 60 will experience occasional impotence.

Cancers of the bladder, colon and

prostate also have been known to cause impotence, as have multiple sclerosis, spinal lesions and some back, head and groin injuries. About 600,000 men are impotent because they've suffered devastating blows to the hidden arteries of their penises—many of them while bike riding, says Irwin Goldstein, professor of urology and co-director of the New England Reproductive Center at the Boston University School of Medicine.

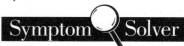

We could bore you with more baseball analogies, but we're going to the bullpen for relief instead. Here's how to treat impotence.

Forgo the fling. If faithfulness to the one you love isn't enough to keep you out of the arms of another, consider embarrassment. Bedding that stranger is far more likely to end in impotence than in sexual conquest.

"This happens more often than we might realize," says Wayne Hellstrom, M.D., associate professor of urology at Tulane Medical Center in New Orleans. "It's usually attributed to having too much to drink or being a little nervous before the affair."

A lurid rendezvous has a way of subconsciously activating the body's fight-or-flight response. This diverts blood from your penis to your circulation and, more often than not, leaves you limp, he says.

Keep on keeping on. If you just lost your membership in the 100 percent club, relax. "It's normal, and you should not be overly alarmed about it," says Dr. Hellstrom. Worrying about the situation can lead to performance anxiety—the dreaded and potentially endless cycle of not being able to get it up precisely because you're worrying about whether you *can* get it up.

Say Yes to Yohimbine

Although the most powerful aphrodisiacs are almost certainly looks, money, power and fame, some experts believe that the bark of an African tree has sexual bite.

Called yohimbine, it's one of the few purported love potions that actually seems to pass scientific muster. In one double-blind study, 450 men took 43 milligrams of yohimbine hydrochloride (Yocon) a day. Within six weeks, 30 percent reported that their erections returned. Not surprisingly, they also reported that their self-confidence improved, says Jacques Susset, M.D., a clinical professor of urology at Brown University in Providence, Rhode Island, and the study's author.

Although more research needs to be done, Dr. Susset says that yohimbine probably stimulates neurotransmitters in the brain, causing erections and increased libido.

Still, yohimbine has gotten a bad rap because most of the preparations on the market don't seem to work, says James P. Goldberg, Ph.D., a clinical research pharmacologist in San Diego and co-author of *Sexual Pharmacology*.

Only the synthetic version, known as yohimbine hydrochloride, has been proven reliable in scientific studies, says Dr. Susset.

There are three synthetic versions that your doctor

"In rare circumstances you may have to visit a counselor or sex therapist to see if there's anything deeper at work, but you probably just need to relax and let things happen," he says. You'll probably be relieved to find that your erection reappears after you stop focusing on your failure.

Limit the booze. You may feel like a sexual Superman after having a few drinks, but it appears that prolonged heavy drinking may can prescribe for you—Yocon, Yohimex and Aphrodyne—says Varro E. Tyler, Ph.D., professor of pharmacognosy at Purdue University School of Pharmacy, West Lafayette, Indiana. But those who do get their doctors to write a prescription often don't use it long enough to get results.

"The problem is that doctors don't tell their patients that they need to take it every day, three times a day for at least four weeks before it will work," Dr. Susset says. Dr. Susset, himself, has taken yohimbine eight times a day for ten years without any side effects, he says. However, he says that about 24 percent of patients cannot take yohimbine in any dose because they may experience some side effects.

Dr. Tyler, in his book *The Honest Herbal*, asserts that yohimbine "dilates blood vessels of the skin and mucous membranes."

Side effects, according to Dr. Tyler, include anxiety. Yohimbine should be avoided by those suffering from diabetes, hypotension and heart, liver and kidney disease, he cautions. An additional note of caution: Yohimbine is a monoamine oxidase inhibitor, which means that aged and fermented foods, as well as nasal decongestants, should be avoided.

process when the liver is damaged by long-term alcohol abuse, he says.

Kick those butts—quickly. The sexual health of some men may literally be going up in smoke—thanks to their cigarettes. That's because smoking causes something called vasoconstriction.

"When you take a puff on a cigarette, the distance between the two walls of your blood vessels narrows," says Dr. Burman. "Over time, the amount of blood that travels through there is diminished. It has a very marked, very pronounced and very well-known damaging effect on your blood vessels."

Although there's no evidence that quitting will reverse the damage, it should halt the decline, he says. As if you needed more motivation to kick those butts quickly, one expert says that smoking has been linked to impotence in 35-year-old men.

Cap that cholesterol. Men with a total cholesterol level over 240 are nearly twice as likely to suffer from impotence than their health-conscious brethren with readings under 180. If the warnings about cholesterol's link to common men-killers such as heart disease and stroke don't scare you, this should. Simply put: If you want to continue having sex, you need to lower your cholesterol count. The best way to achieve that goal is to eat less fat, eat more fiber and exercise at least three times a week, say nutrition experts. You may even try supplementing with garlic, a proven cholesterol cutter. "In our studies, we are finding that when subjects take nine garlic capsules per day—each capsule containing 800 milligrams of dry garlic extract—their cholesterol decreases 8 percent after four months," says Yu-Yan Yeh, Ph.D., professor of nutrition at Pennsylvania State University in University Park. Each capsule

turn a so-called man of steel into a paper tiger. "More research needs to be done, but it's just very common to see people who've had severe alcoholism come into our center with impotence," says Jack Jaffe, M.D., medical director of the Potency Recovery Center in Van Nuys, California. "My feeling is that it causes damage to the blood vessels of the penis." Not only that, but testosterone remnants are broken down in the liver, which may interfere with this is about the eqivalent of one clove of garlic. If this seems like too much garlic even for a true garlic-lover, don't fret. Dr. Yeh says that even a small amount—two or three cloves a day—may help lower cholesterol.

Work it out. Regular exercise does more than just help keep your veins and arteries clear and keep the weight off. It also gives your self-image an important boost. "The way that you look in the mirror is going to make a difference as to how you feel about your sexual performance. If you look good and you feel good about yourself, you're going to come on more aggressively, more strongly and with a greater sense of confidence. The chances of your failing are going to be correspondingly less," says Dr. Burman.

Think zinc. Though not an accepted treatment by most mainstream urologists, there is some evidence that zinc is linked to potency. That's because zinc helps your testes create testosterone, the male hormone that, among other things, helps you maintain normal muscle mass and sperm levels. The candidates most likely to benefit from a zinc supplement are those men with moderate to severe zinc deficiencies, says Curtiss Hunt, Ph.D., of the U.S. Department of Agriculture–Agricultural Research Service at the Grand Forks Human Nutrition Research Center in North Dakota. And this group may be getting bigger all the time. In the quest to shed fat, many men are shunning red meat, one of the best dietary sources of zinc. Other good sources of zinc are seafood (especially oysters), pumpkin seeds, whole-grain cereals and legumes. A three-ounce serving of lean ground beef provides roughly one-third of the 15 milligrams of zinc you need each day. A cup of raisin bran provides up to 10 milligrams of zinc.

Give prostaglandin a shot. Do you

Pump It Up

What feels like the real thing, looks like the real thing and, unlike the real thing, is good for hours of enjoyment? The penile implant.

Thanks to the wonders of modern medicine and advanced technology, it's now possible to get it up and keep it up—long after most regular guys have fallen flaccid.

"You could even say that a penile implant is better than normal," says Dr. Sheldon Burman of The Male Sexual Dysfunction Institute. "A regular man goes soft after he comes. Patients who have a penile prosthesis can have sexual intercourse all day, all night and the next day if they want to," he says.

In one such operation, doctors insert two thin, long, spongy cylinders into your penis. Next, they insert a small saltwater reservoir behind your pubic bone on top of your bladder. Finally, they insert a grape-size pump into your testicles.

remember the biochemical prostaglandin E_1? Although it's found naturally in your body, doctors have discovered that injecting some into your penis allows the smooth muscles to relax and blood to flow there—just like the real thing.

If you've only experienced impotence on occasion, chances are that your doctor may give you an injection in his office just to show you that your vascular mechanisms that cause an erection still work. Within 10 minutes you should have an erection that lasts anywhere from 30 minutes to an hour. "When you look down and see that you have an erection, it gives you the kind of reassurance that can be very beneficial," says Dr. Hellstrom.

If you've had more frequent bouts, your doctor may suggest that you be placed on a

Then, according to Dr. Burman, when it's time to have intercourse, you gently—and we mean gently—squeeze the pump in your testicles, which fills the cylinder with water, which gives you an erection "as big and as fat and as hard as you had when you were 17."

After performing more than 1,700 such operations, Dr. Burman says that he's never had to remove one because of a mechanical malfunction. The most common complication that he's encountered, seen in less than 2 percent of patients, involves a few very overweight men with diabetes who developed infections.

Medicare statistics show that of every 1,000 men getting a noninflatable penile prothesis, 103 will later need an operation to correct a complication. Of every 1,000 men getting an inflatable penile prosthesis, 227 will later need an operation to correct a complication. Complications usually involve either the breakdown of the device itself or infection, which can happen with any surgery.

cise, eating lots of whole grains and vegetables, and possibly helping to stabilize your blood sugar by using supplements like chromium and vitamins B_6 and B_{12}, says Dr. Hellstrom. The Daily Value for chromium is 120 micrograms, 2 milligrams for vitamin B_6 and 6 micrograms for vitamin B_{12}. If impotence does come, however, it's not the end of the world. You're a likely candidate for a PEP, pharmacologic erection program, like prostaglandin shots or another form of treatment, says Dr. Hellstrom.

Patch it up. Men diagnosed with low testosterone levels should get a boost from prescription testosterone patches on the market. "Testosterone is related more to libido than impotence, but it will help men who have impotence because of low testosterone," says Phil Hanno, M.D., professor and chairman of the Department of Urology at Temple University School of Medicine in Philadelphia. Counting your chest hairs won't tell you your testosterone level; you'll need to see your doctor.

self-injection program using the prostaglandin E_1 shot (also known as Caverject) at home. A training session follows that includes how and where to perform the injection, says Dr. Hellstrom.

Experts claim that the injections are successful in 70 to 80 percent of patients, although some complain of burning or pressure after the injection. Since in rare cases it's also been found to cause blood clotting, experts also don't advise using Caverject on cruises or trips out of the country, says Dr. Jaffe.

Deal with diabetes. Unfortunately, most experts feel that it's inevitable for men suffering with diabetes to become impotent. But you may be able to slow the decline by arresting your diabetes. Strategies include getting your weight under control through exer-

Get pumped up. Depending on your attitude toward sex toys, an at-home treatment called vacuum therapy could become the most fun you've had with a small appliance. Consider this: First you cover your penis with lubricant. This helps create an airtight seal when you place your penis in the special vacuum's cylinder. Using a small pump, suction power then helps draw blood into your penis, creating an erection. Finally, rubber rings are placed at the bottom of your penis to make sure the blood stays there. (Experts caution against using the rings for more than 30 minutes at a time.) Don't be fooled by cheap imitations that you find advertised in the back of magazines. You'll need a doctor's prescription to buy a real one—and some instructions on how to work the darn thing—before you're ready to go.

Low Sex Drive

- You're spending more time with Frank Gifford than with your partner
- You've noticed a dramatic decline in sexual interest

What It ? Means

Life is full of cruel ironies. In college, you majored in couch wrestling. But when the love of your life cornered you near the dishwasher last night—in that pouty, amorous way of hers—all you could think about was, "Doggone it, I'm going to miss Monday Night Football!"

Don't sweat it. While it's true that you're supposed to have a fairly strong sex drive—or libido—until late in life, nearly every guy goes through times when his interest in sex takes a backseat—even to key televised NFL showdowns.

But if she's been chasing you at all hours—without success—for a few weeks now, you could be suffering from low libido: a dramatic, though far from permanent, pause in your level of passion, says Miriam Baker, Ph.D., staff associate in the sex therapy program at New York Hospital-Cornell Medical Center in New York City.

"You don't feel attracted to anything. Nothing stimulates your interest. You lose your fantasy life. There's an immediate or slow decline in your sexual interest—in every way. There's just nothing happening," she says.

Sound familiar? You're not alone. "I'd say that at least 80 percent of men at one time or another undergo some kind of serious, temporary change in their interest in sex," says Stanley H. Ducharme, Ph.D., a health psychologist in the Department of Urology at Boston University Medical Center.

The Lowdown on Low Libido

Two of the most common causes of low libido are depression and sexual problems such as impotence or premature ejaculation. "If the whole sexual experience has a hint of frustration, failure or feelings of inadequacy associated with it, then that will translate into low libido," Dr. Ducharme says. Relationship problems are another obvious cause, he says.

Some antidepressants and high blood pressure medications are hidden causes of low libido. In fact, antidepressants such as fluoxetine hydrochloride (Prozac), paroxetine hydrochloride (Paxil) and sertraline hydrochloride (Zoloft) are so effective at putting the brakes on your sex drive that they're used for other sexual dysfunctions as well. "We have actually revolutionized the area of treatment for premature ejaculation with these medications," Dr. Ducharme says. (Before you stop taking any medication, talk it over with your doctor.)

Excessive work, hobbies or other interesting or important projects—like keeping up with league standings—have been known to temporarily reduce interest in sex. "Take exercise. You feel good about yourself—not in a direct sexual way, but it provides you with some of those positive measures of self-esteem. If this is the source of your problem, it's something that you don't need to worry about. You'll snap out of it soon enough," says Dr. Ducharme.

If you've checked none of the above so far, there's a remote chance that you're suffering from low testosterone. Like high-octane fuel, testosterone is the male hormone that keeps your sex drive humming. Without the right amount of testosterone coursing through your system, you're likely to keep the car in the garage, so to speak.

It's unlikely, however; only about 2 percent of all men suffer from low testosterone, says Dr. Jack Jaffe of the Potency Recovery Center.

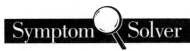

Unlike some sexual problems, there are plenty of simple things that you can do to help give your libido a lift. Here's how it's done.

Make yours yohimbine hydrochloride. Often prescribed for impotence, this synthetic version of an African tree extract could be just the pick-me-up your dwindling libido needs. In fact, one researcher who studied yohimbine treatments for impotence says that men who weren't even complaining of libido problems got a boost.

"Though there was no super effect above and beyond normal, they showed, if anything, more improvement in libido than erection," says Dr. James P. Goldberg, a clinical research pharmacologist and co-author of *Sexual Pharmacology.*

To get results, you must use yohimbine for at least four weeks, "and you should notice an effect between three and six weeks," says Dr. Goldberg. Yohimbine apparently stimulates testosterone-sensitive areas of the brain, he says.

It is important to note that yohimbine is a monoamine oxidase inhibitor, which means that aged and fermented foods, as well as nasal decongestants, should be avoided. Also, the herb should not be taken by people with diabetes or heart, liver or kidney disease. Check with your doctor if you want to try this therapy.

Get wowed by Wellbutrin. It's sold by prescription as a nonaddictive antidepressant, but experts say that bupropion hydrochloride (Wellbutrin) offers tremendous hope for those suffering from low libido.

"The effect is gradual, like working out, but in cases where you just don't seem to have the sexual energy, it could bring you back to where you were in your teens and early twenties," says Dr. Goldberg. During one study of 60 men and women who suffered from a lack of sexual desire or sensation—but not depression—Dr. Goldberg says that he found that "Wellbutrin specifically decreased or eliminated their sexual problem."

Unlike most other antidepressants, which stimulate serotonin and essentially relax the individual, Wellbutrin apparently stimulates dopamine in the brain, which helps increase sexual interest. "It's almost in a class by itself," he says, particularly since the serotonin effect of other antidepressants may decrease sexual interest and response.

Talk it out. The last thing that most guys want to do when they have a problem—especially with sex—is to talk it over with someone else.

Big mistake.

"Men tend to close themselves off to the resources available to them and go inward. But the most effective way to deal with depression—and that's often at the root of low libido—is to get some emotional support," Dr. Ducharme says. "Telling someone that you have this kind of problem should not be seen as an emasculating experience. It's very important for men to realize that this is a common problem. It doesn't mean that you're any less of a man."

Avoid anti-fantasies. If your low libido has its root in dissatisfaction with your mate, you might be able to shift your sex drive out of neutral by focusing on your partner's best qualities. "You have the option of drawing on the positive aspects of her and the relationship or the negative or what we call anti-fantasies," says Dr. Baker. "Ask yourself, 'Am I going into this sexual situation only thinking about my partner's anti-fantasies, anything that is not sexy, or good-quality, stimulating fantasy material?' If you are dwelling on the bad stuff, you're resisting feeling sexual, and that's going to cause problems."

Put the real in relationships. Is standing in line at a convenience store your idea of getting close to someone? You may be using your low libido as an excuse to remain emotionally distant from your partner.

"Often this is used to avoid vulnerable intimate situations—either physically or emotionally. You're shielding yourself, preventing yourself from getting into a vulnerable emotional situation. Learn to get closer, or get some help doing it," says Dr. Ducharme.

Give yourself some time. Folks who have gone through serious psychological trauma like a huge breakup, separation, divorce or death deserve a few months to recuperate.

"A lot of people who complain to me about impotence or lack of libido have just been through one of these kinds of problems. I've seen it often enough to believe that it's a common self-protective mechanism," Dr. Ducharme says. The worst thing that you can do when you're in this situation is to jump from one relationship to the next.

"The healthy thing is to take a few months and kind of get your feet back on the ground—restore your stability. When you really feel safe again, that's when you can get close." If the withdrawal persists beyond several months, you may need to seek professional counseling.

Take a hormone test. No Number 2 pencil is needed—just the willingness to give a little blood to your urologist. From this simple procedure, he'll be able to see whether your testosterone level is where it ought to be, says Dr. Phil Hanno of Temple University School of Medicine.

Pick your treatment. If your testosterone level is low, you used to have a choice between a patch worn on your dry-shaved scrotum or periodic testosterone injections. But now, a new patch—a testosterone transdermal system called Androderm—can be applied nightly on the abdomen, back or upper arm.

One study showed that 92 percent of

Key Questions

To help identify the source of your low sex drive, therapists suggest that you ask yourself a few penetrating questions (and answer them honestly).

- Is this problem truly a sexual disorder, or is the sex problem really a consequence of other issues in my relationship?
- Is it mainly a problem of differences in desire between my partner and me?
- Are either of us taking some medication that might be to blame?
- Is the decreased desire actually secondary to some other sexual disorder (for instance, erection problems or pain during intercourse)?
- Is it she who doesn't turn me on, or do I have trouble getting aroused by anyone? (If it's only she, you're likely to have relationship problems.)
- If I increased my interest in sex, what bad things might happen?

---

men who used Androderm saw that their testosterone levels were steadily boosted. The most common side effect is skin irritation at the application site.

Dr. Jaffe, however, offers these words of caution: "In my view, testosterone should only be used as you would prime a pump—just a little to get it started." His recommendation is to receive injections of long-acting testosterone every one to two weeks for four or five times only. If that's unsuccessful, your doctor may refer you to another health professional for treatment.

See a pro. When your low libido includes loss of energy, fatigue, lack of initiative, insomnia or loss of appetite, you may have a more serious problem on your hands—like depression. "These are indications that people should consider some professional intervention," says Dr. Ducharme.

Premature Ejaculation

• You're not lasting as long during sex as you—or, perhaps, your partner—would like

What It ❓ Means

Let's face it guys: If many of us aren't careful, sex can be a lot like the Super Bowl. You know the experience: weeks of intense preparation, media interviews and posturing by the participants. Anticipation builds to a feverish pitch. The whistle blows. And . . . the game is over by the end of the first quarter—leaving even the most loyal of fans frustrated and disappointed.

But don't pack up the pom-poms quite yet. (Especially if your partner is about to do that cheerleader thing.) Sex doesn't have to be that way—even for the most frequent premature ejaculator, says Dr. Miriam Baker of New York Hospital-Cornell Medical Center. Although not a health problem, premature ejaculation can be caused by conditions such as stress or impotence. But often, it's just a matter of learning to control your sexual sensations.

"It takes some patience and practice to learn how to handle yourself in bed, but just about anyone can do it," she says.

Symptom 🔍 Solver

Want to know how to keep the play spirited until the final gun sounds, so to speak? Here are some ideas that can help.

Bag the trick plays. When trying to delay orgasm, some guys use what could be called a diversionary tactic. They think of pass completion averages or yards per carry. Or even football's Dallas Cowboys guard Nate

Newton dressed up in drag—anything to keep them from ejaculating too soon. This kind of approach is not only unreliable; it does not fix the problem and can lead to problems in the long term.

"When you get older and your erections aren't quite as easy to come by, if you lose an erection, you then focus on getting it back, which adds another problem—and both problems remove you from the pleasure of your sexual experience," Dr. Baker warns.

Rate your arousal. Like pro scouts, sex therapists have their own rating system, but *theirs* is for arousal. A zero, of course, is a zero, while a ten is certainly a touchdown, two-point conversion included. Before you start pushing eight or nine on the arousal scale, Dr. Baker says that it's time to back off a little. "You don't want to zip all the way to a nine and just hope for the best. But six or seven is a good place to be for as long as you can. You'll want to remember what that feels like so that you can do it again," she says.

Go to the running game. You're willing to slow the tempo, but how? Stop trying to throw the long ball. "You stop stroking your partner or thrusting so much. Just hang back a bit and relax," Dr. Baker says. "Learn that if you just kind of close your eyes for a minute, let the feeling trickle backward and stop moving in a less orgasm-directed way, very quickly the sensation abates. Before you know it, you're at a six."

Master the moment. You gave it your best, but now you're wiped out and she's still ready, willing and virtually begging to play. At this point, most guys just limp to the sidelines and settle for a warm place on the bench.

But you can stay in the game. In fact, if you come out with a few innovative plays and are still willing to execute, you might end up a most valuable player in her eyes. Just because you're tired doesn't mean that your arms and hands are broken. If your orgasm has happened before hers, you can assist her pleasure before rolling over and falling asleep, Dr. Baker says.

Semen Problems

• Your rifle's cocked, but it's shooting blanks; no sperm in your semen

• You've noticed a change in the color or smell of your semen

• You see blood in your semen

What It ✌ Means

We've been told that we're not sensitive enough. (Compared to whom? Phil Donahue?) Forgetful. (What do you mean this is the second anniversary of our third date?) And now this: We're not the men that our fathers were.

That nervous buzz that you hear is the collective concern of fertility experts poring over data that suggest a worldwide drop in sperm count and semen quality. At last glance, the average Joe had a sperm count of 66 million per cubic centimeter of semen. According to statistics, his fedora-wearing counterpart in 1940 cranked out nearly twice as many. For the record, if your sperm count falls below 20 million, you're thought to have reduced fertility; a 5 million count means that you're sterile.

To be sure, not everyone agrees that we have big-time semen quality problems. In fact, some experts suggest that it might simply have to do with improved accounting procedures.

But even if you're inclined to blame the guys with the calculators, it's hard to ignore the observations of Earl Dawson, Ph.D., associate professor in the Department of Obstetrics and Gynecology at the University of Texas Medical Branch at Galveston and the author of several fertility studies. "We're located here in Galveston, and we get medical students from all over the state. And when you see one of these hot-blooded, 22-year-old freshman medical students come in here from Longhorn Springs, in west Texas, where he has lived all his life on beef and beans and has never come in contact with venereal disease or anything like that, and even he has a low sperm count, you begin to understand that this may really be something happening worldwide."

Rounding Up Suspects

Possible suspects depend on the researcher. Some point to increased chemicals in the environment acting like estrogen—the hormone that produces breasts and other interesting characteristics in women. Others suggest toxicity from industrial pollution in the form of lead, aluminum, carbon dioxide and many others. But in Dr. Dawson's view, the main problem is lead. "It doesn't have a taste, it doesn't have a flavor, but it's in the air, the dirt, the dust," says Dr. Dawson. "They've taken sophisticated vacuum cleaners out in the streets and found lead on the side of the roads. Remember the big unleaded gas push years ago? That's why we had to remove it. Evidence has shown that lead is toxic to damn near anything. And I have found it in seminal plasma and found it strongly associated with decreasing sperm viability."

And if some kind of environmental toxin isn't damaging your sperm, maybe your old sports injury is responsible. In a study by the University of Wisconsin Medical School of 179 infertile men, researchers found that those who reported testicular injuries from sports such as football, bicycling, wrestling and martial arts had a 25 percent higher level of a female hormone in their bodies than those who couldn't recall an injury. Secreted after testicular trauma, the hormone is believed to decrease or impair sperm production, according to researchers.

Ironically, of less concern is blood in your semen. In older men, it can be a symptom of cancer. But it most cases, blood in your semen is usually caused by a broken blood vessel or an infection, says Dr. Jack Jaffe of the Potency Recovery Center.

An orgasm that does not produce ejaculate can be a warning sign for diabetes, experts say. Clear ejaculate might mean that your seminal vesicles aren't pitching in when they should. However, a little early morning clear urethral discharge is common in younger men and not a cause for worry. Yellow ejaculate may mean that the opening of your bladder isn't closing tight enough to prevent urine from leaking in. Although not harmful to your health, it may reduce sperm quality. If your semen is yellow and smells bad, you could have a urinary tract infection. For any of these, see your doctor.

Symptom Solver

Although your efforts to produce progeny have yet to meet with success, experts say that it might just be a matter of making small changes. Try these tips.

Let OJ save the day. Based on both research and anecdotal evidence that he's observed during his career, Dr. Dawson says that he would instruct his own son to drink a quart of orange juice every day to boost his sperm count. "I've gotten letters from men around the world who had read of my research work. A few read something like this: 'My wife and I have been trying to have a child for five years. I went into training for something or other and started drinking orange juice every day as part of my training program. All of a sudden, my wife got pregnant. After I read the newspaper story about your work, I realized that it was the orange juice that I was drinking that made me more fertile.' And so this is why I say to drink a quart of orange juice a day," says Dr. Dawson.

Try vitamin C and see. In addition to orange juice, Dr. Dawson recommends 500 milligrams of vitamin C, both in the morning and with dinner, for two weeks, and then 500 milligrams per day. A water-soluble vitamin—which simply means that you'll urinate it away once the body has enough—vitamin C

apparently protects sperm against toxins like lead and nicotine. In one study, Dr. Dawson divided 75 young male smokers into three groups. One group got a placebo, another got 200 milligrams of vitamin C daily for a month, the third took 1,000 milligrams of vitamin C each day for a month. Also, the higher the men's vitamin C levels rose, the greater the protection they received against the sperm-damaging effects of nicotine.

Drink more milk. The ads say, "Milk, it does a body good." If Dr. Dawson is right, they aren't kidding. "I think the main idea is to get the Daily Value of calcium because calcium will also inhibit lead," he says. In the days when paint contained much more lead and before other treatments were found to reduce lead poisoning, doctors would actually prescribe a quart of milk a day to painters who developed lead poisoning, says Dr. Dawson. The Daily Value of calcium is 1,000 milligrams. Two glasses of skim milk and a cup of low-fat yogurt is all that it takes.

Eat more zinc. Men who eat less zinc than recommended have less ejaculate, according to a study authored by Dr. Curtiss Hunt of the U.S. Department of Agriculture–Agricultural Research Service at the Grand Forks Human Nutrition Research Center. As zinc intake fell from more than 10 milligrams per day to just above 1 milligram, the amount of ejaculate dropped by nearly one-third. Although his study didn't measure fertility, Dr. Hunt says that it's bound to be affected somehow. Found in lean beef, crabmeat and oysters, the Daily Value of zinc is 15 milligrams.

Slip into some boxers. Although the evidence isn't, shall we say, rock solid, some experts suggest that wearing boxer shorts can help improve fertility by keeping your testicles cooler. "The idea is that testicles are normally outside the body, and if they are pulled up closer to the body, the excess heat will make a difference," Dr. Jaffe says. Heat may decrease the amount of sperm produced.

Testicular Lumps

- A lump of any size on the otherwise smooth, even surface of a testicle

- Enlargement of the testicle

- A dull ache in the lower abdomen or groin

- A sudden collection of fluid in a testicle or in the scrotum

- Pain or discomfort in a testicle or in the scrotum

What It Means

There are a couple ways to check for testicular lumps. You could wait until you're hit in the crotch with a baseball—à la former Philadelphia Phillies first baseman John Kruk—to become generally more aware of what's happening down there. Or you could use the method preferred by the National Cancer Institute: a monthly, one-minute testicular self-examination starting at age 15.

Frankly, we prefer the second technique. Not only is it less painful, but it also seems to be more effective. As you may recall, Kruk had to have one of his testicles removed. And he was fortunate. "We've seen guys wracked with advanced testicular cancer because they've ignored testicle lumps for several months or even years," says Judd Moul, M.D., a urologic oncologist in the Department of Surgery at Walter Reed Army Medical Center in Washington, D.C., and director of the Center for Prostate Disease Research at the Uniformed Services University of the Health Sciences in Bethesda, Maryland.

Fortunately, testicular cancer is rare; only about 3 men in 100,000 per year contract it. But what it lacks in frequency, it makes up for in precision: Testicular cancer is the most common form of cancer among guys between the ages of 15 and 35.

Doctors haven't been intimidated, however, and within two decades have gone from a 10 percent cure rate to nearly 100 percent when the disease is caught early.

Unlike other cancers, testicular cancer doesn't seem to be linked to any of the usual health abuse suspects, like smoking, alcohol or fat. Instead, experts theorize that there are three links: one genetic, another as a result of a decreasing size of the testicles from mumps or a virus, and the third related to an unusual condition found in some male babies who have had undescended testicles.

About the time that you were born, your testicles were supposed to have dropped from inside your body and find their home in your scrotum. But if they didn't drop before age six, a doctor probably came looking for them—with a surgeon's knife. Despite successful surgery, experts have observed that men who had undescended testicles as boys are 3 to 17 times more likely to develop testicular cancer. (If you're a dad with a young son, you might have your son examined by a pediatrician to be sure that the testicles have properly descended.)

If you had undescended testicles, there's a good chance that your parents told you about them or that you noticed a scar that led you to ask. You may have even been taught how to check for testicular cancer. If not, it's you and the rest of the guys living in moderately blissful ignorance that we're worried about. Because, frankly, this is one health problem that you don't want to ignore. "Testicular cancer is one of the most aggressive cancers. The growth rate is very high, so we consider it an urgent situation when a young man discovers a testicular lump. We get on it immediately," says Fuad Freiha, M.D., professor of surgery and chief of urologic oncology at Stanford University.

The most common way that testicular cancer is discovered is during a warm shower, which apparently relaxes your scrotum and allows you to feel any irregularities more easily. "In the great majority of cases, a young man walks into the office and says, 'I was showering yesterday and felt this mass in my testicle,' " says Dr. Freiha.

What if that happens to you? First, make sure that you haven't discovered your epididymis—a cord-like structure to the rear of each of your testes. (They're supposed to be there.) When in doubt, see your doctor.

Be on guard for any testicle pain and swelling, a lump in either testicle, a feeling of heaviness in your scrotum, a dull ache in your lower abdomen or groin, or enlargement or tenderness of your breast—also symptoms of testicular cancer, says Dr. Freiha. (For more on that, see "How to Perform a Testicular Self-Exam.")

Then visit your doctor, says Dr. Freiha. If he's suspicious, he'll perform an ultrasound scan to determine whether further treatment is needed. If cancer is discovered, the entire testicle—and any other affected tissue—is almost always removed. (Even if you have a testicle removed, you'll still produce semen when you ejaculate; however, your sperm count probably won't be as high as it was, unless your other testicle is normal.)

During the operation, the surgeon will not cut through your scrotum or the cancerous testicle because cancer cells can spread. The cut will be in the inguinal region or groin. Surgeons will often remove lymph nodes deep in your abdomen to learn whether testicular cancer cells have spread.

While surgery certainly isn't something to look forward to, it is highly effective, relatively uncomplicated and has few side effects other than discomfort (one of the more common is numbness on one side of the scrotum, which generally clears within six months).

If, however, the malignancy has spread to lymph nodes in the abdomen or, worse, to

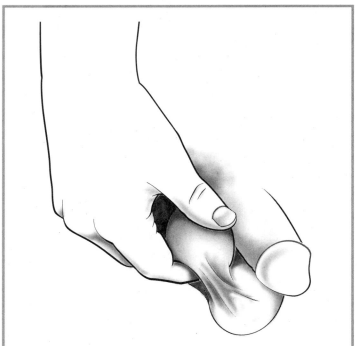

How to Perform a Testicular Self-Exam

1. Grasp each testicle between your thumb and first two fingers.

2. Gently run your fingers around the circumference of each testicle, feeling for any lumps or hard places. The testicle should have the feel of a small hard-boiled egg without its shell.

At the back of each testicle, you'll find a cordlike structure called the epididymis. It belongs there. The rest of the surface should be smooth and rubbery. If you find a lump of any type anywhere, see your doctor immediately. Also, call your doctor if you feel any soreness or swelling.

the lungs, follow-up treatment—ranging from radiation to chemotherapy to a second surgery—may be needed. It depends on the nature of the tumor and how far it has spread.

Although the options sound grim, it should be noted that the disease is highly responsive to the weapons used against it.

The key is to catch it early, and the most effective way to do that is a regular testicular self-exam.

Urination Problems

- You have a slow urine stream

- You experience a burning sensation when urinating

- You awaken several times in the night to urinate

What It ? Means

Remember those peeing contests that you had with your buddies when you were a kid? The ones that determined your place in the neighborhood pecking order by just how far you could let it fly?

Of course, we've outgrown such childish notions. Today we know that there are better gauges of true manhood—like what kind of car you drive, for example. Okay, so maybe we haven't outgrown all our childish notions. But it turns out that the way we urinate can tell us quite a bit about our health, if not our machismo.

"Difficulty urinating, a slow stream, burning while you urinate, getting up several times a night to urinate—these are all changes in your urinary habits that you need to pay attention to," says Dr. Judd Moul of Walter Reed Army Medical Center.

Here's why. When you're young and healthy (not to mention full of your favorite beverage), urine flows from your kidneys and into your bladder, a balloonlike muscle that expands as it fills. Upon reaching capacity—and finding the nearest bathroom—your urine is ready for its a downward descent.

To picture what happens next, imagine a straw pushed an inch or so through the hole of a mini-doughnut. Urine flows through the straw, called the urethra, past the doughnut—

actually a walnut-sized gland known as your prostate. It's a quick trip from that portion of your urethra—which runs the length of your penis—and out of your body.

Unimpeded, your urine stream is long and strong—good enough for a first-place ranking on that good old neighborhood scale—and an A-plus from your urologist.

On the other hand, a faltering stream can signal some potential health problems. In fact, it's such an important clue that most urologists start checking you out by having you answer a small battery of questions related to urinary habits and their effect on your quality of life. Among other things, their inquiring minds want to know whether your bladder ever feels full after you've urinated and how often you have to go again less than two hours after you've already gone.

Livin' Large

One of the most common causes of these kinds of urination problems in men age 50 and over is benign prostatic hyperplasia (BPH)—in other words, an enlarged prostate. By itself, an enlarged prostate isn't a big deal. Unfortunately, as the prostate grows, it can put the squeeze on your urethra. "The main symptoms of this would be a slowing of the stream and having to wait for the stream to get going," says Dr. John Mulcahy of Indiana University Medical Center.

But the fun doesn't stop there. Thanks to the blockage, your bladder has to squeeze even harder to eliminate urine, potentially increasing the number of times that you feel like you have to go to the bathroom. As a result, urine can stagnate in the bladder, causing infections. You might even see blood in your urine—often the result of blood vessels in your prostate or bladder that have burst. "The worst thing about BPH isn't the fact that your prostate is enlarged but how much that enlargement is interfering with the quality of your life," Dr. Moul says.

Frequent urination or pain when you urinate can also be caused by what's called prostatitis, a catchall term used to describe an infection or inflammation of the prostate. Prostatitis can also block urine flow resulting from prostate swelling, causing a backup that can lead to bladder or kidney infections. How would you know if you had prostatitis? This ailment comes complete with additional symptoms such as pain between the scrotum and rectum, fever and pus or blood in the urine. And those of us who can't seem to keep it in our pants may want to pay special attention: One of the most common causes of prostatitis is chlamydia, a sexually transmitted disease (STD).

Another STD—gonorrhea—and some medical treatments, such as a prior cystoscopy or a catheterization of the urethra, can scar your urethra, which can also slow your stream or cause pain when you urinate. Gonorrhea is almost always accompanied by a thick, yellowish discharge between urination.

An inflammation of the bladder lining called interstitial cystitis has been linked in some rare cases in men to an increased need to urinate and burning while urinating.

The patriarch of all prostate problems, prostate cancer, can also cause changes in urine flow. But if you're under age 50, relax; chances are good that you don't have it.

When suffering from urinary problems, however, it's probably wise to pay a urologist a visit—regardless of your age. By the time you notice any other symptoms—like low back pain—the cancer may have already spread. "The American Cancer Society and the American Urological Association, recommend that men start getting checked for prostate cancer at age 50. However, for African-American men and men who have a family history, it's recommended that they get checked once a year starting at age 40," Dr. Moul says.

During your visit, your doctor will gently examine your prostate for hardness, lumps and bumps—all telltale signs of cancer, says Dr. Moul. Roughly 10 to 20 percent of all men with BPH may have prostate cancer.

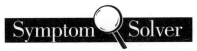

The causes are many; fortunately, treatments aren't few. Consider these helpful tips for urinary problems.

Be berry merry. Saw palmetto berry, that is. Long considered a home remedy for BPH, European medical studies seem to show that this herbal treatment has some basis in scientific fact. During one French study, for example, 94 men with BPH took either saw palmetto extract or a placebo. Within a month, the men taking saw palmetto had increased flow rate, visited the bathroom fewer times at night and lessened urine remaining in the bladder after urination by 42 percent.

How does saw palmetto work? Scientists say that it may prevent the breakdown of testosterone into dihydrotestosterone, a more potent form of the hormone that researchers believe may cause prostate enlargement. It may also serve as a mild anti-inflammatory, thereby helping shrink the prostate. Those who advocate saw palmetto for BPH also say that it has no side effects—unlike prescription BPH treatments, which can cause low libido, impotence, dizziness and breast enlargement.

Give smart cycling a try. No need to trade in your bike for a treadmill. Experts say that you can avoid aggravating your prostate while bike riding by making some simple changes, says Dr. Mulcahy. You can start by ditching that narrow, there's-no-way-my-butt's-gonna-fit-on-that Italian racing seat for a softer, wider model. Then make sure that the seat tilts forward slightly and raise your handlebars. Sitting on the horn of the seat long-term can inflame the prostate.

Use a condom. The most common urinary problems among young men are caused by STDs, says Dr. Jack Jaffe of the Potency Recovery Center. Most can be avoided by using a condom.

Try zinc to shrink. Although controversial, some doctors believe that zinc deficiencies are linked to BPH. In one of the few scientific studies that tested the theory, 14 of 19 men who took zinc supplements saw their prostates shrink in two months. "It has been implicated to have a role in prostate health for many years, and some patients swear by zinc supplements," says Dr. Moul. "I think that there might be some value in zinc. We need more good-quality studies to evaluate it in a scientific fashion."

Ironically, in the quest to shed fat, many men are shunning red meat, one of the best dietary sources of zinc. Also found in oysters, lamb, whole-grain cereals and peanuts, the Daily Value for zinc is 15 milligrams. How much is that? Two steamed oysters would put you well over the top.

Watch these foods. There are no known food causes of BPH, but several can irritate your bladder lining. This seems to aggravate an enlarged prostate, leading to urinary problems.

Most experts recommend avoiding caffeinated beverages, alcohol (including beer and wine), tomato and tomato-based products, spicy foods, fruit and fruit juices, milk products, sugar, honey, corn syrup and artificial sweeteners for seven to ten days. If your symptoms go away, you've found your culprit. "For some men with mild symptoms, adjusting their diets may improve their quality of life and prevent the need for other treatment," says Dr. Moul.

Delete the decongestants. Over-the-counter nasal decongestants like Sudafed may slow your runny nose, but they also wreak havoc on urine flow. "These have the effect of tightening a belt around the prostate, resulting in slower urination," says Dr. Mulcahy. Some doctors recommend them for incontinence, the involuntary leaking of urine from the bladder.

Prescribe relief. Prescription drugs like tetrazosin hydrochloride (Hytrin) and doxazosin mesylate (Cardura), which are muscle relaxers, have been found to relax the neck of your bladder, allowing urine to flow more freely, Dr.

Trickle-Down Theory

It never fails. You stop in the men's room to relieve yourself before the big presentation, and just as you're tucking yourself back in your pants, one last squirt trickles out on your trousers.

Embarrassing? Absolutely. Annoying? Most definitely. Avoidable? Read on.

Make room. Pull your pants far away from your penis, and don't try to urinate by pulling your penis over the top of your underwear. Use your fly. That's what it's there for. By not giving your penis enough room to urinate, you slow the flow of urine through your urethra, the small tube that expels urine. As a result, urine that isn't expelled dribbles out when you tuck yourself away.

Milk it. After you finish urinating, apply some gentle pressure behind your scrotum with one hand and coax out any remaining urine. This is where the widest part of your urethra is, the part where urine tends to pool in men. Gentle pressure might be all that you need to get rid of those last few drops.

Mulcahy says. "If you're getting up three or four times a night to go to the bathroom, treatment with one of these may allow you to get up once or not at all," says Dr. Mulcahy.

See a surgeon. As a last resort, your doctor may suggest that you have surgery—an operation one doctor candidly described to us as a "roto-rooter." During the operation, doctors will trim the prostate tissue that's blocking the flow of urine through your urethra. Be aware, however, that a small percentage of men have suffered sexual dysfunction and scarring of the urethra as a result of these kinds of operations. "Before you have this done, you should always get a second opinion after trying the more conservative treatments or medications without success," says Dr. Mulcahy.

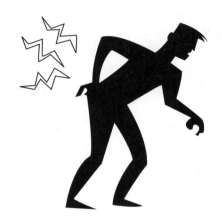

Part Six

Arms, Legs and Back

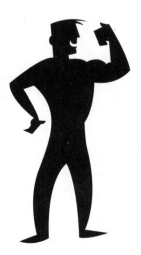

Ankle Pain

- Your ankle is painful and/or swollen after a twisting injury to the foot

- You have pain when standing, with a sense of instability

What It Means

Until we actually have 500 cable channels, you'll probably never see an international competition to determine the most commonly sprained joint. No matter. The ankle already wins—feet down.

Any sport that requires quick stopping and starting—be it basketball, racquetball or tennis—is notoriously tough on the intricate ankle joints. Even a casual jog on uneven pavement can be enough to turn your ankle, tearing the inside or outside ligaments that help hold the entire structure in place, says Donald Baxter, M.D., president of the Orthopedic Foot and Ankle Society and an orthopedist in Houston.

Just make sure that your ankle pain is caused by a sprain. "Ten to 20 percent of ruptured Achilles tendons are missed because people think that they have a sprain," says Saul Trevino, M.D., of the American Academy of Orthopedic Surgeons and clinical professor at Baylor College of Medicine in Houston. One easy but potentially painful way to find out: Gently stand on your toes. If you feel like someone just ran your calf through a meat grinder, you have a torn Achilles tendon. If not, it may be your ankle after all.

For a possibly less painful test, Dr. Trevino suggests that you have someone gently squeeze your calf to see if the injured foot moves in a downward direction. If it does, the Achilles tendon is not ruptured, although it could still be injured to some degree.

It may seem obvious, but a once-sprained or a once-fractured ankle that heals improperly is another common cause of ankle pain, says Dr. Baxter.

Making the Grade

Bony impingements, nerve compressions, arthritic spurs—even arches that are too high or flat—are other possible causes of ankle pain, Dr. Baxter says. But the dreaded sprain is so common that it has its own grading system.

A grade-one ankle sprain is the least severe—it doesn't hurt immediately. In fact, you may not even see any swelling until long after you've hit the showers.

Although it may not cause the most pain, a grade-two sprain can actually be the most troublesome. "These are the ones that swell up immediately," Dr. Baxter says. "But because they're only a partial tear, often the ligaments are so stretched out that they never heal back nice and tight." Like a bent rim on a bike, the weakened ankle is susceptible to future breakdown.

A grade-three sprain can make the blowout of a steel-belted radial tire look pretty. The upside is that it has good healing potential. "It's probably black and blue, you can't walk, everything is ruptured, but if you wear a brace or some other kind of immobilization for a while, it can heal back tight," Dr. Baxter says.

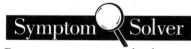

By now, most guys who know their way around a locker room know that R-I-C-E spells relief from ankle pain. Well, not literally. It actually stands for rest, ice, compression and elevation. But you have to do the RICE combination right to get results.

"It's just not enough to wrap the ankle, place your foot in a bucket of ice and expect to get better," Dr. Baxter says.

Depending on the extent of the injury, rest could very well mean between three days and two weeks of performing some kind of exercise that's less stressful to your ankle. Ice should be wrapped in a towel and applied for 15 to 20 minutes a time at least three times a day. Proper compression involves wrapping an elastic bandage loosely around your ankle but with some type of pad—like a folded washcloth—placed directly on the injured area. And don't forget elevation—this also helps reduce swelling. Just make sure that you raise your ankle above your heart—your toe should be as high as your nose, says Dr. Baxter.

But here are some new twists on ankle pain treatments you can try.

Keep your shoes on. Friends have told you this to save their noses; an expert tells us that it can help prevent swelling and decrease healing time of a sprain. "Trust me . . . if you took the shoe off, your ankle would puff up, and you would not get your shoe back on. But if you keep it on, it keeps the swelling down," says Garry Sherman, D.P.M., a former team physician for World Team Tennis now in private practice in Cedar Knolls, New Jersey. Dr. Sherman advises that you keep your shoe on until you get home and are able to apply the RICE method, or—if you think there is a fracture—until you get to the hospital.

Test your ankle awareness. What were you doing just before you heard that awful popping sound? And how were your feet positioned? You may be trying to block out the accident, but remembering how your injury occurred can help to speed healing and give you a quick way to decide whether to seek treatment, says Dr. Trevino. Turning your ankle in—roughly what happens when you place your shoes sole to sole—is usually far less severe than turning your ankle out.

"If you turn your ankle out, you'll probably have some tendon damage or a possible fracture, and you need to be much more concerned about that. You should probably see a doctor," Dr. Trevino advises.

Engage in four-play. If your swelling and pain are nearly gone, you should begin rehabilitating your ankle on the fourth day, says

Dr. Sherman. This would include taking short walks, massaging and kneading your ankle and doing exercises like drawing circles in the air with your toes. If your pain recurs, stop the activities.

"You don't want to overdo it, but you've got to start motion immediately," he says. "The longer you are off that foot and keep it inactive, the more scar tissue you develop. And the more scar tissue that develops, the worse your recovery is going to be. Sometimes you can even get permanent loss of motion."

Other simple ankle strengtheners include two sets of calf raises three times a week (20 reps each set) done by simply going up on your toes, walking on your heels for 1½ minutes or picking up marbles with your toes.

Pack some heat. After three days of ice, heat will help your rehab by drawing fluid to your ankle and keeping it loose, Dr. Sherman says. Applying a hot-water bottle or heating pad 15 minutes before you exercise your ankle should do the trick, he says.

Air it out. Can't sit out any more games this season? Try an air cast. "That's what athletes use, and they're right back on the field in three days. While it may feel awkward, it both supports your ankle and prevents it from turning," says Dr. Sherman. Air casts cost about $50 and can be purchased from most medical supply stores.

Get examined. If immediately after the injury you can't stand at all on your foot or if you're not walking in a week, there's a good chance that you need to see a doctor. And pay attention to bruising or new popping noises. "If your ankle pops when you turn it, that's probably when you need to be evaluated by a physician," Dr. Baxter says.

And if you have your ankle x-rayed, at least one expert says that you may want to schedule another appointment. "If it's an out-and-out break, it will show up right away," Dr. Sherman says. "But if you have any question in your mind, it's also a good idea to have an x-ray ten days later."

The problem, Dr. Sherman says, is that a fracture will not necessarily show up on the initial x-ray. "If you keep walking on it, a hairline fracture will get worse and turn into an overt break," he warns.

Turning Things Around

To avoid future injury, try these tips.

Achieve a proper balance. No surprise here, but folks who are agile are less likely to suffer serious ankle sprains than those who can't walk and chew gum at the same time, experts say. If you seek medical treatment, chances are that your physical therapist will train you on what's called a balance board—a computerized board that helps to improve your agility.

Don't want to go that route? Practice on your own. "It sounds kind of silly, but you can practice maintaining your balance by standing on one leg. It's basically the same kind of exercise, and it works," says Dr. Trevino. If that's too easy, try it with your eyes closed.

Wrap it up. Having your ankle taped does provide some support, but after 10 to 15 minutes, Dr. Trevino says, the tape often stretches, reducing the benefit. As a result, some experts recommend ankle wraps made from leather or other materials that are designed with the frequent ankle sprainer in mind. Costing between $50 and $150, "these provide tremendous support and will allow someone who has had major ankle difficulties to compete again," says Dr. Trevino. The sturdier wraps are only available through your doctor.

Try some high-tops. Here's more ammunition to help justify those high-priced high-tops. Experts say that they might help prevent ankle pain. "The nerves around your ankle feel the pressure of the high-top, so you react a little bit more toward the variations of the terrain," Dr. Baxter says. "The friction or the pressure of the high-top on the ankle allows you to better sense where your foot is. You're less likely to turn it. They also provide support."

When researchers compared the rate of twisted ankles among men who wore shoes cut above the ankle and men who wore below-the-ankle models, they found that the high-tops provided almost a third more protection. The researchers note that there's a split second after your ankle starts to collapse, but before leg muscles can catch it, when support from a high-top shoe can help.

Strive for golden arches. Whether you have flat feet or super high arches, you might be able to relieve the ankle pain that they cause by being fit for an orthotic device. Placed in your shoes, orthotics help your feet achieve the optimal arch for your foot. "This brings the foot in better alignment, which can eliminate bone pressure on the outside of the ankle and eliminate ankle pain," says Dr. Sherman.

It's probably best to talk to your doctor about the orthotic that's right for you. Although an inexpensive, over-the-counter orthotic device could work just fine, there's a good chance that it won't. "Unfortunately, many over-the-counter orthotic devices are made for people whose feet are inclined to turn inward. If you try one on and it doesn't feel right, don't try to wear it anyway. You may have the wrong one," says Dr. Sherman.

Hang loose. Tight Achilles tendons can make wearing your orthotic device painful. Here's an easy stretch for keeping them loose, says Dr. Sherman: Step forward with one foot, resting your hands against a wall. While keeping your hands on the wall, keep your rear foot flat and your leg straight and lean against the wall, stretching one leg at a time and holding for a count of five. Repeat with the other leg.

Try a little tendon-ness. Tendon strength is the key to avoiding ankle sprains. So Carol Frey, M.D., chief of foot and ankle surgery at the University of Southern California Medical School in Los Angeles, recommends the following exercise. Sit and loop a towel over the top half of your foot. Apply resistance by pulling your leg upward while you push your foot up and down. Try three sets of 20 reps.

Arm Pain

- You haven't had your arm twisted in years—and it still hurts or goes numb

What It Means

If you're experiencing arm pain, the list of potential suspects narrows rather quickly. Bad training habits at the gym can cause bicep pain. Pain from repetitive-motion injuries like carpal tunnel syndrome can start in your wrist and radiate up your arm. Neck and nerve strain can take the other approach, shooting pain down your arm.

If you think that your arm pain might be caused by carpal tunnel syndrome, see Wrist Pain on page 122. If you suspect that it might be originating from your neck, see Neck Pain on page 118.

But there's another potential cause of arm pain and weakness that, though a little bizarre-sounding, may be worth a closer look.

Nerves and veins travel from your neck to your arm through something called your thoracic outlet. (This is the area just behind your collarbone.)

But in a chest breather—someone who doesn't take full, deep breaths—the scalene muscles (normally used for deep breathing) in his thorax flex when they aren't supposed to, squeezing both nerves and veins in the thoracic outlet. This, in turn, causes pain, numbness and weakness in the arm and hand—a condition that doctors have dubbed thoracic outlet syndrome.

"I've seen the worst of the worst cases—people who have often had multiple surgeries to try to fix their arm pain—and more often than not, they have a problem in the thoracic outlet," says Peter Edgelow, a physical therapist and co-director of Physiotherapy Associates in Hayward, California.

Symptom Solver

If you've been unable to find fixes for the arm pain that you suspect is related to thoracic outlet syndrome, try this tip.

Make your belly dance. Although it's still a controversial theory, Edgelow and some other medical professionals believe that you may be able to relieve some of your arm pain or numbness by learning how to breathe with your belly (diaphragm) rather than with your chest (scalene muscles). Lie down on the floor with your knees comfortably bent, and put one hand on your stomach and the other on your chest. Try to lift the hand on your stomach by taking a deep breath and expanding your stomach like a balloon that is being blown up. The hand on your chest should stay still. As you breathe out, let your belly contract and gently blow the air out through pursed lips. Repeat for three minutes and then as often during your day—without lying down—as possible.

Edgelow has worked with more than 600 patients suffering from severe neck and arm pain and believes that relearning the proper breathing technique is essential to relieving their pain. "I teach them to pay attention to their tension and blow it away."

For combating other types of arm pain, here are two additional suggestions.

Clean up your curl. A small number of men suffer arm pain because they're twisting their wrists while they do bicep curls, says Darryl L. Kaelin, M.D., medical director of Outpatient Rehabilitation Services for Community Hospitals of Indianapolis. Instead of twisting your wrist all the way forward when curling, keep it straight, he says. Switching to an E-Z curl bar—a curling bar that has angled sections for gripping that help keep the wrists in their proper position—also will help, he says.

Take a break. It should be common sense, but if your arm is causing you pain, doctors say that the smartest thing to do is to rest it for a few days.

Back Pain

- You have low, mid- or upper back pain

- You hear Michael Jackson's "Bad" every time you think about your back

What It Means

Every guy would like to think that he has some "MacGyver" in him. The TV saint of resourcefulness, each week our hero would be forced to escape from some deadly predicament using little more than a common household object. Thermonuclear device about to detonate? No problem! MacGyver pulls out a lint brush and goes to work.

Nothing, however, quite deflates that can-do spirit like back pain—especially low back pain, far and away the most common back complaint. When the ache sets in, most of us would just as soon slouch around in our bathrobes for weeks on end than do anything heroic—or anything at all, for that matter.

And yet, experts say that long-term inactivity is among the worst ways to treat back pain. After more than just a few days off your feet, the very muscles that are struggling to keep your spine in line lose even more strength, setting you up for future pain, says Stanley Bigos, M.D., chairman of the U.S. Public Health Service's Agency for Health Care Policy and Research panel on back pain, a group of 23 health care specialists, headquartered in Rockville, Maryland, who studied traditional back pain treatments. "We've learned the hard way that the best thing for back pain is not to take it easy at all unless absolutely necessary."

But if resting on your backside isn't the best way to treat back pain, what is? Maybe staying moderately active *and* watching the calendar. Experts say that in nine out of ten cases, the pain simply goes away in about a month. "I think that sore backs have a lot in common

with colds," says Peter Slabaugh, M.D., an orthopedic surgeon in private practice in Oakland, California. "They're two of the most common afflictions known to mankind—nearly everyone suffers from back pain at least once by age 50. And we've come to realize that in most cases, back pain just runs its course with no long-term damage."

Even back pain that radiates down your leg doesn't cause the red alert that it once did among doctors. "Roughly 25 to 40 percent of all back patients will have some leg pain. Now if you also have bowel and bladder disorders, severe weakness or have trouble walking, you'll need to see a doctor," says Dr. Bigos. (Falls and car crashes that cause back pain or back pain with fever or chills also require an office visit.)

In fact, you need to be downright wary of doctors who feel a need to name your back pain. "Our research shows that 88 percent of the time, doctors call it a sprain, strain, myofascitis, disk syndrome, internal disk derangement or degenerative disk disease, but what they really mean is, 'I don't know,'" says Dr. Bigos. "Less severe back problems often defy diagnosis."

On balance, however, the inability to make a specific diagnosis for lesser back problems is a plus, says Dr. Bigos. "We can skip the abstractions and zero in on the important things, like what you are asking your back to do and what kind of condition you keep yourself and your back muscles in," he says. It's also making doctors less likely to recommend surgery. Research by the panel that Dr. Bigos chaired shows that only 1 in 100 back pain sufferers benefit from going under the knife.

Of course, if your symptoms persist for more than a month, it may be a good idea to see a doctor after all to find out why you are in the slowest 10 percent to recover.

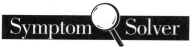

And the rest of us inactive action heroes? Although high-tech solutions for our back pain are limited, there are plenty of quick and easy ways—even if we're just slightly resourceful—to make ourselves more comfortable and avoid future pain.

The pain just flared, and you're ready for relief. Here's how it's done.

Do a little power lounging. Normally associated with munching chips or hanging out at the beach, the official power lounging position— knees slightly bent and body reclined as if in a chaise lounge—is the best way to relax while your back mends. "Of all the positions, this takes the stress off the low back the best, even better than being flat on your back," says Dr. Slabaugh.

Get back on ice. You can apply ice wrapped in a towel to a sore back if it makes you feel better, especially for upper back and neck pain. "At minimum, 15 minutes before you go to bed, just after you get up in the morning and at least one other time during the day should help a lot," says Dr. Bigos. "If your symptoms are bad enough, keep applying ice for three to five days."

Get down, but not for long. As we already mentioned, the days of languishing for weeks on end developing your Oprah IQ are gone. But how much time should you take off to recuperate? As a rule of thumb, figure on the same length of time that it took Nick Nolte and Eddie Murphy to hash out their problems on the big screen: 48 hours. That, of course, can vary "depending on the kind and extent of your injuries," Dr. Slabaugh adds.

Quit yer sittin'. If you think that you're doing your back a favor by sitting in that straight-back chair, think again. "Studies show that sitting is the most stressful position for your back, especially when there is pain. And frankly, people don't think of that because they think, 'I'm resting my back and legs.' But they actually could be prolonging the problem," says Dr. Slabaugh.

Going Both Ways

Switch-hitting has always been a valuable skill in baseball. Sometimes it causes confusion in the opposing team's outfield or knocks its pitcher off stride long enough to drive in the winning run.

But at least one doctor believes that a form of switch-hitting when you run or play golf or tennis may be useful for keeping your back healthy.

The idea is simple: The next time you line up for a shot or practice swing, try one with the opposite hand. In theory, this opposite-handed rotation will run counter to the normal rotation, helping prevent muscle strain, says Joseph Askinasi, a member of the American Academy of Sports Medicine and a chiropractic orthopedist in New York City. "If you are a runner, try walking backward on a track for a lap or two. This should also be of benefit," he says. "I have recommended this to my back pain patients for years—and with great success."

Give your knees a lift. Some experts suggest sleeping with a pillow under your knees to keep them elevated. This may remove some stress from your lower back. For relief when you're sleeping on your side, place your pillow between your knees, says Dr. Bigos.

Do an NSAID. That's nonsteroidal anti-inflammatory drug to you, pal—like ibuprofen. But you may want to talk to your doctor about taking a higher-than-normal dose. "To get the anti-inflammatory effect in an average-size man, I'd say that he should take three capsules three times a day—and that's a smaller dose than when we're writing a prescription," says Dr. Slabaugh. Because NSAIDs can cause gastric upset when taken on an empty stomach, use them with food.

Have a belt. Your weightlifting belt is a lot cheaper, and perhaps more comfortable, than the corset that a doctor is likely to insist that you wear. "Wearing a weightlifting belt while you're still in pain holds up the weight of your body. And the more of your body that it holds up, the less that your spine has to do," Dr. Slabaugh says. "A weightlifting belt can also pull your stomach in a little bit and flatten out your swayback, putting your back in a much less stressful condition while you're recuperating." What's more, wearing a weightlifting belt limits your ability to stoop and bend, reducing pressure on the disks of your spine, he says. That's why it makes sense to wear one when you're lifting heavy objects.

Allow yourself to be manipulated. You may not care much for office politics, but manipulation—the kind that chiropractors, massage therapists and osteopaths perform on your spine—has been found to provide about the same relief from back pain as ibuprofen or acetaminophen. "If you can control your symptoms with this and stay active, you're way ahead of the game," says Dr. Bigos. If your symptoms don't improve within a month, however, get another opinion.

Hang with a TENS. It sounds like a relic from the East German Olympic training program. But a transcutaneous electrical nerve stimulator—a TENS unit, for short—is designed to zap fast-twitch muscle fibers, helping to stop spasms and reduce your pain. Although research results on the TENS are mixed, many people swear by them, says Dan Spengler, M.D., professor and chairman of the Department of Orthopedics and Rehabilitation at Vanderbilt University Medical Center in Nashville. Some chiropractors, osteopaths and family doctors have TENS units.

Get moving. Low-stress exercises such as walking or swimming are an excellent way to help get your back into gear, while minimizing further injury, says Peter Edgelow of Physiotherapy Associates. "The heart and the physical movement of your body pump your circulation, and this promotes healing," he says.

Avoiding Back Pain

To head off back pain in the future, consider these tips.

Build your back muscles. Pumping iron in the gym may help you build bulging

Back Relief

While lying on your back, bend the leg on the painful side so that your foot is flat on the floor and as close to your buttock as comfortable.

Ask a friend to grasp the thigh that's in the air just above the knee and pull it away from your body as if to make you longer. Repeat this action up to ten times, first gently stretching and then releasing. Do not continue if it increases your pain. This position can reduce the stress from your lower back, providing immediate relief.

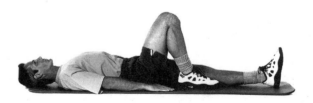

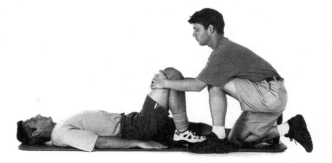

biceps, but all that you may need to condition your protective back muscles is a pillow and a place to lie down. (See the illustration of this back-strengthening exercise on page 108.)

Sound too simple? Consider the results of a Swedish study involving 60 nurses with back problems. The group was divided in half: 30 performed the same back exercise each day; the rest didn't. After two months, researchers discovered that the exercisers had one-tenth as many back complaints and one-fifth the number of days lost because of back problems as the nonexercisers, Dr. Bigos says. The exercise strengthens the erector spina muscles—those that run right next to the spine along the back.

Tone your trunk. There's less agreement about the role that your abdominal muscles play in keeping your back healthy. But some doctors say that even swinging a tennis racket or hitting a golf ball can be downright dangerous to your back if your trunk is weak. "These sports require a lot of twisting of the torso, and you need to have those muscles of the abdomen and the back extensors in shape so that you can handle that," says Dr. Spengler.

One of the best ways to build trunk strength is weight machines at the gym. "Use anything that has weights and a pulley—like a Nautilus machine—so that you can measure your progress," says Dr. Spengler. Other doctors recommend performing three sets of crunches (where you lie on your back with your knees bent and slowly curl your upper torso until your shoulders leave the floor) every other day to help strengthen abdominal muscles.

Shape up. Keeping your whole body fit may be one of the best ways to keep your back free from pain, Dr. Bigos advises. "Just 30 minutes a day, speed walking, cycling or jogging helps condition your muscles, your entire body,

---

The Arnica Advantage

Need to be kneaded when your back is acting up? Are you a sucker for salve? Then you'll love arnica.

Made by crushing a flower and soaking it in alcohol, arnica was discovered by Europeans in the late sixteenth century and perhaps earlier by the Native Americans. With documented anti-inflammatory and analgesic properties, arnica is so popular in Germany that it's used in more than 100 different healing products there. It has been reported that massaging with commercially available arnica tincture reduces pain and swelling of bruises, sore muscles and sprains—common causes of back pain. Be aware that there is a compound in arnica that can cause contact dermatitis in some people. (Contact dermatitis is a skin rash that can include itching, swelling, blistering, oozing and scaling.) The application of arnica should be stopped immediately if such a reaction occurs. In addition, tincture of arnica is for external use only.

---

to better tolerate those little stresses that can cause big problems," he says.

Drop those pounds. "It's really easy to understand. If you have a stomach that sticks out, it just puts that much more stress on your lower back," says Dr. Slabaugh. Eating less fat, and getting your 30 minutes of aerobic activity three days a week should help you shed pounds, he says.

Support your local lumbar. Be they rolls, pads or cushions used in your chair or car, studies show that you can decrease the stress on the lower back by using lumbar supports. And that means that you'll stay comfortable longer. Lumbar supports are available at many drugstores and medical supply stores.

Butt out for good. Smoking not only

reduces the benefits of aerobic exercise—stamina—but is also probably bad for your spine. "Let's face it, most people who smoke have a tendency not to do things to keep their aerobic activity high," says Dr. Spengler. "But the research has also clearly shown that smoking adversely impacts the spine."

Be suspicious about stretching. Until your body is completely warmed up with at least several minutes of light exercise, some doctors say that you should avoid stretching. "Think of your back as a chain of vertebrae that are linked together by a joint. As with a chain, when you stretch a chain, you are only stretching the weakest link. So it's not too surprising that stretching can irritate the spine," says Dr. Bigos.

Be a clock watcher. Even the fittest desk jockey with a history of back pain can suffer if he doesn't give his back a periodic break, Dr. Spengler says. Consider standing or taking a quick stroll down the hall every hour just to put your back in a different position.

Bounce that billfold. It's probably not a major cause of back pain, but sitting on your wallet can push your pelvis out of alignment, or press on your sciatic nerve, potentially causing pain.

"I've never seen any scientific studies on this, but it makes sense. When I get in the car, I just kind of instinctively take my wallet out and put it somewhere because it makes me more comfortable," Dr. Slabaugh says.

Give yourself the chair. There are chairs, and then there's the chair. If you're going to be sitting anywhere for vast stretches of time, make sure that your chair has these features: a firm seat, a back that comes up to at least mid-shoulder level, armrests, built-in lumbar support and a slight backward tilt—between 5 and 7 degrees, says Dr. Slabaugh. "It would be great if you could tell people to get a new job where they don't have to sit all the time. The best that you can do is modify the environment as much as you can," he says. If your chair is for home use, add a footrest that keeps your knees slightly bent.

Get your feet fixed. Maybe improper foot alignment is causing your back problems. The theory goes something like this: If you pronate when you walk or run—that means that your heels are slightly falling to the side—this may rotate your knee and, as a result, affect your posture.

How would you know if your feet are improperly aligned? Dr. Garry Sherman of Cedar Knolls, New Jersey, suggests standing directly in front of a full-length mirror after a shower. If your knees point inward or outward instead of straight ahead and your hips and shoulders appear uneven, you should probably see a podiatrist about your foot alignment. In one study, among those fitted with custom orthotics designed to address their pronation, 77 percent of the patients showed a 50 to 100 percent improvement in symptoms. The rest reported 25 to 50 percent improvement.

Back Builder

Place a pillow on the floor and lie facedown on top of it, resting your pelvis on the pillow.

Use your back muscles to lift both of your legs and your chest slightly off the floor, but keep your back bowed no more than when standing. Keep the back muscles tense as long as possible, until you can hold the position for four minutes before you go to bed each night.

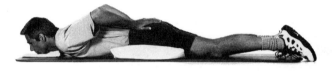

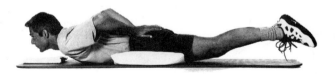

Elbow Pain

- Dull, persistent pain in your elbow
- Swelling

What It 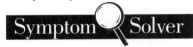 Means

Even if your command of physics comes from watching *Beakman's World* with the kids on Saturday mornings, it's not hard to figure out why tennis players suffer from elbow pain. A just-belted tennis ball travels at about 100 miles per hour. A swiftly swung racket clocks in at about 180 miles per hour. During the course of a two-hour match, tennis ball and racket—held in place by your meager arm—collide over and over again. The result is microtrauma at the most vulnerable point, usually the tendons and ligaments of your elbow.

Microtrauma—literally microscopic tears—doesn't seem like it would cause big pain. But combine it with the inevitable tendon degeneration that sets in as we reach our thirties and forties and you have elbow problems, says Gerald R. Williams, M.D., co-director of the elbow and shoulder service at the University of Pennsylvania in Philadelphia.

But elbow pain isn't limited to only those who bat a fuzzy green ball around. In fact, 95 percent of those suffering from elbow pain picked up their ailments at work. Often these are folks who perform repetitive arm movements: assembly-line workers, meat-packers, computer typists, even carpenters.

Still, these cases often feature the classic tennis elbow symptoms: dull, persistent pain and possibly swelling of your elbow for 6 to 12 weeks. Even shaking hands hurts.

Other Causes

Another possible source of elbow pain is called ulnar nerve compression—essentially a pinched funny bone. Although not nearly as common, this symptom seems to affect baseball pitchers, some racket sports players and again, some occupations such as assembly-line workers and computer typists.

Duffers have their own version of elbow pain, called, appropriately enough, golfer's elbow. Apparently, overusing the trailing right arm by pushing the club through (for those who swing right-handed) can overload some slightly different muscles, causing pain.

And don't forget the elbow leaners. These are the guys who routinely strike the thinking man's pose and, if they thought better of it, could easily avoid elbow pain. "It sounds funny, but if you do it often enough, leaning on your elbows can cause irritation of the ulnar nerve," Dr. Williams says.

Arthritis and gout also can set up shop in your elbow, causing pain, while carpal tunnel syndrome has been know to radiate all the way to the elbow. (For more information on carpal tunnel syndrome, see Wrist Pain on page 122.)

As far as tennis elbow and golfer's elbow are concerned, you don't have to be a scientist to understand that some people simply have more durable tendons than others. "It's like this: Some are born with 20,000-mile tires, and others are born with 60,000-mile tires," says Robert P. Nirschl, M.D., director of Virginia Sports Medicine and Rehabilitation Institute in Arlington and associate clinical professor of orthopedics at Georgetown University in Washington, D.C. "Either way, you can't really trade them in. You just have to make them last the best way that you can."

Symptom Solver

Since you probably don't want to give up tennis—or other activities that cause elbow pain—you can learn to minimize the ache. Sure, doctors say that you can take an over-the-counter nonsteroidal anti-inflammatory like ibuprofen before or after your activity to help ease the pain. But keep in mind, says Dr. Nirschl, that these medicines only comfort; they do not cure. You can also try these tips.

Brace yourself. For about $20, you can buy a double-strap, contoured Nirschl Counter Force brace or a single-strap model that offers less muscle support. A brace may help reduce elbow pain—regardless of whether you play tennis. "Worn on the forearm, it helps to decrease the tension generated by the muscle, thereby protecting the tendon," says Dr. Nirschl, creator of the brace and co-author of *Arm Care: A Complete Guide to Prevention and Treatment of Tennis Elbow.* More expensive straps featuring fluid- or gel-filled pads can concentrate pressure, which may frustrate normal balanced muscular strength, he says. For more information on Nirschl Counter Force braces, you can call 1-800-783-2240.

Stretch smartly. You can maintain flexibility by stretching before work or tennis, Dr. Williams says. Extend your right arm in front of you until your elbow is straight. With your palm down, slowly bend your wrist until your fingers are pointing toward the ground. Using your left hand, gently press the top of your right hand until you feel a tension stretch at the top of your forearm. Without any movement, hold for 15 seconds. Repeat with the other arm.

Now extend your right arm in front of you with your palm up. Using your left hand, gently press as if you wanted to push your right wrist down. But don't move the arm. Hold for 15 seconds, applying steady pressure. Repeat with the opposite wrist. This exercise stretches the bottom of your forearm.

Call on the curl. One of the best exercises for helping to strengthen the muscles susceptible to elbow pain is the wrist curl, says Dr. Nirschl. Take two light dumbbells (or a barbell) in both hands and sit down on the edge of a bench, knees close together. Rest your wrists on your knees so that your hands are hanging off (palms down). Keeping your wrists on your knees and forearms on your thighs, curl the weight up and down for three sets of 15 reps.

Put the hammer down. Hammer twists are another effective exercise for strengthening forearm rotation and preventing elbow pain, says Dr. Nirschl. With your left hand, grab a hammer at the very end of its handle and sit with your elbow propped at the very end of a table. (Place a towel or another type of cushion under your elbow to soften the surface of the table.) Keep your wrist straight, allowing your forearm to hang off the edge of the table. Now slowly rotate your hand from side to side as if you're pouring a glass of water. Repeat with the other hand. Work up to three sets of 16 to 20 repetitions.

Give a squeeze. Here's another way to strengthen the muscles that fend off elbow pain, says Dr. Nirschl. In each fist, squeeze a tennis ball or a wad of rolled-up newspaper 25 times, holding each squeeze for three seconds. Repeat this two more times and continue the routine every other day.

Get a grip. Simply changing grip sizes up or down seems to reduce tennis elbow pain for some. "The most important thing is to find a grip size that's optimal for you," says Dr. Williams. (Don't feel left out if you use hand tools. The same wisdom may very well apply. Try it and see, he advises.)

Dr. Nirschl adds that it is probably better to err on the side of a bit bigger grip in order to control torque. A grip that is too small can be trouble, he says.

Don't get framed. Metal tennis frames are notorious for transferring force from impact with the ball to your elbow—a perfect setup for tennis elbow. Instead, choose a composite frame—they're designed to absorb the impact, says Dr. Williams.

Loosen up. Tennis strings too tight? They're another possible cause of tennis elbow. "The looser the strings, the more impact that the strings absorb and the less that your arm absorbs. The tighter the strings, the more energy that gets transferred down your arm and into your elbow," says Dr. Williams.

Knee Pain

• You're not just weak in the knees, but sore, too

What It ✷ Means

There were times when it seemed that he would never make it to the huddle. Just watching Joe Namath—brash, cocky, swaggering Broadway Joe of the upstart Super Bowl champion New York Jets—hobble painfully onto the football field was enough to make a generation of sports fans wince. His knees paid the price for the violent game that he loved. And like another great New York sports idol, the late Yankees legend Mickey Mantle, his marvelous Hall of Fame career ended with wistful questions of what further wonders might have been witnessed if he hadn't been cursed with those bad wheels.

The talent and genius that they brought to their chosen sports may have been uncommon, but the health problem shared by Namath and Mantle is anything but uncommon. Roughly 50 million Americans suffer from knee pain. Torn cartilage is thought to account for about half of that misery. Normally acting as a cushion to help absorb your weight, your meniscus cartilage floats between your thighbone and shinbone like a gigolo between girlfriends—until it compresses between them and tears.

"Squatting in a catcher's position, even a movement as simple as squatting down to tie your shoe or to put air in your tires, can make it happen," says Terry Whipple, M.D., clinical associate professor of orthopedics and rehabilitation at the University of Virginia School of Medicine in Charlottesville and an orthopedic surgeon with Tuckahoe Orthopaedic Associates in Richmond, Virginia. "As you approach 40, these tears tend to occur from fairly innocent maneuvers."

Causes of Pain

Since younger guys move and groove with seemingly reckless abandon, they're more prone to tear knee cartilage while engaged in activities that require twisting or pivoting—like taking the ball to the hoop or rounding first base. Accompanied by swelling, these tears cause persistent pain on the inner side of your knee—especially when you climb stairs. Severe cartilage damage has even been known to make your knee lock.

"One of the pieces of the cartilage gets wedged or jammed between the leg bone and shinbone—like a rug getting caught under a door—blocking the free movement of the knee. The larger the tear, the more likely that the machinery will jam," Dr. Whipple says.

The machinery of the knee is fairly simple. It's held together by tough ligaments that connect, protect and stabilize the joint; cartilage that cushions the bones and tendons that join muscles to bone.

Torn and sprained ligaments, another common source of knee pain, are mainly a younger man's injury. The main reason is that ligament injuries are usually suffered by those participating in various sports like football where guys are knocking heads and bodies. But slip on some ice, wreck your car or smash into a wall while playing racquetball and you may suddenly find that you have more in common than you'd like with those competitive younger men, says Dr. Whipple.

And if that's not bad enough, even mildly damaged cartilage and ligaments often develop bursitis or arthritis. "Cumulative trauma—anything that dents, crushes or chips the cartilage—can lead to arthritic changes," says Dr. Whipple.

If any of this sounds familiar and your pain has persisted for a few days, the best thing that you can do is visit a knee specialist. Without treatment, you're risking permanent damage. (Most sports medicine doctors know knees well; you'll find them listed in the phone book in most major metropolitan areas.)

Generic knee soreness, caused by things like too much running or wrong exercise technique, is another matter. Kneecap pain, for example, known by the guys in the white lab coats as patellofemoral pain, makes its presence known either when you're climbing stairs or when you're forced to sit in one place for a long time, says Edward R. Laskowski, M.D., co-director of the Mayo Clinic Sports Medicine Center in Rochester, Minnesota. Often a result of tight tissue on the outside of the thigh, in combination with a weak inner thigh muscle, this condition causes the kneecap to track to the outside, irritating underlying tissues and causing pain.

Hauling around that paunch isn't exactly doing your knees a favor either. Experts say that being overweight is another common cause of knee pain.

Vitamin C to the Rescue?

If your knee pain is caused by the early stages of arthritis, grab a bottle of orange juice—not a rocking chair. Research hints that vitamin C may slow the disease before it slows you.

In a Boston University study of 640 people with and without knee osteoarthritis, those with the highest vitamin C intake had three times less disease progression than people with the lowest intake of that vitamin (less than 120 milligrams a day—the amount in two average oranges).

The results suggest that this group lost less cartilage and was likely to develop less pain during the eight years of the study than did those who didn't get that nutrient. Some people high on the scale of dietary vitamin

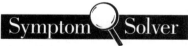

Though knee injuries can be serious, there are plenty of ways to provide quick relief or prevent them. The basic formula for acute joint injuries holds especially true for knees, says Dr. Whipple: Do RICE—rest, ice, compression and elevation. Get off your knee for a few hours. Pack some ice wrapped in a towel on the swollen area and leave it on for no more than 30 minutes every hour. To elevate your knee properly, make sure that your toe is higher than your nose. "It's not the cure, but it will help you feel better. It will help ease your symptoms," says Dr. Whipple. Here are some less familiar—but highly effective—ways to combat knee pain.

Squeeze your knees. Just because knee pain has set in doesn't mean that you have to let your quads and hamstrings wither. Try this exercise: First, roll up a towel or use a pillow and place it under your knee. Then slowly press your knee right into the towel or pillow for three sets of 12 reps with a few seconds of rest between reps.

"This will help to preserve muscle strength in an injured leg if you're not using it that much," says Dr. Laskowski. "Once that's pain-free and comfortable and you have good motion in the knee—you want to have motion before we strength train aggressively—you could probably progress up to doing a leg press, lunge, wall squat or similar exercise."

Make sure that you're riding right. Ordinarily, bicycle riding helps build both muscle and lung capacity without any impact. The perfect exercise for your knees, right? Not necessarily.

"The seat must be set properly. When you're pushing the pedal down, you should have about a 20-degree bend in your knee. If the seat's too low, you may actually cause knee pain," Dr. Laskowski says. Once you're riding right, pedal for at least 30 minutes three or more days a week to help build pain-free knees.

Walk this way. After you've biked comfortably for a few days to help treat your sore

E and beta-carotene also kept their arthritis from getting worse. But those results were less convincing.

The study was too preliminary to draw firm conclusions, but study leader Tim McAlindon, M.D., assistant professor of medicine at Boston University School of Medicine, suspects that these antioxidant vitamins are important when inflammation from arthritis is in full swing. Inflammation is believed to release free radicals that do more damage to the joint—unless antioxidant vitamins are there to stop the radicals from doing harm.

Translation: Antioxidant vitamins may not stop you from getting arthritis. But it's possible that they can stop it from wearing away the joint so quickly.

knees, you may want to try some walking, says Dr. Laskowski. An excellent form of exercise, walking is easy on the joints, while improving aerobic fitness. And in at least one study, researchers discovered that during an eight-week program of supervised walking, folks with arthritic knees had less pain, were able to walk farther and used less medication than those not on a walking program.

"Warming up a joint increases its blood supply, and an increased blood supply makes fluid leak out of blood vessels, lubricating and softening tissues," Dr. Whipple says. "Look at it this way: It's easier to bend a wet piece of spaghetti than a dry piece of spaghetti."

Question leg extensions. They're found in gyms the world over, but some experts are beginning to suggest that using leg extension machines may be linked to knee pain. Unlike a squat or a lunge that distributes weight across muscle groups, leg extensions place a lot of stress and shear force on the knee joint, warns Dr. Laskowski.

"There are some therapeutic and rehabilitative uses for that machine, but our studies have found that the shear force on the knee is actually less when doing a squat or a lunge than when doing a knee extension," he says. "The average person may do more harm than good by using one."

Get a leg up. If you're reluctant to give up leg extensions—or don't think that they're the source of your problem—at least make sure that your leg workout includes other exercises, like leg curls, leg presses, squats and lunges.

"Quads and hamstrings are like guy wires on either side of the knee. If you have one strong guy wire and one weak one, your knee is still in jeopardy," Dr. Whipple warns. "On the other hand, balanced, strong muscles help protect the ligaments, tightening in response to any force applied." Try doing three sets of 10 to 12 reps until you can perform the exercise easily, and then raise the amount of weight that you're using.

Be a flexible guy. Most men scoff at stretching and head straight for the squat rack. But keeping your knees flexible may help keep them healthy and pain-free, says Dr. Whipple. "If you can keep your ligaments and cartilage flexible, they are less likely to tear," he says.

One technique: Stand on your left leg and pull your right heel gently back until it touches your buttocks. Change legs and repeat. "This stretches the quadriceps muscle, but remember: If the muscle isn't well-conditioned, responsive, strong and flexible, then the loads are applied to the ligaments," says Dr. Whipple.

Performed correctly, the stretch helps maintain flexibility of the medial collateral ligament (on the inner side of the knee) on the bent knee and the hamstring muscles of the straight knee.

Act reflexively. Quick reflexes are vital for helping your thigh muscles protect your knees from sudden slips and accidents. "If your muscles don't contract quickly, they play no protective role, and your ligaments get injured," Dr. Whipple says. "If the muscle has fast reflex time—that is, it can contract very quickly—it will better protect the joint as soon as the force is applied."

To improve reflex time, run through tires, skip rope or even have a friend or coach point in different directions as you run toward him, changing direction as he moves his arm. "Reflex training is exactly what it sounds like: You respond or react to some outside source of information," says Dr. Whipple. "You're going to be called on to move in one direction or another, but you don't know which way or when. You always get some of that training by playing sports where you are called to redirect your movement suddenly, like basketball, racquetball or tennis."

Lose the flab. Surgeons are so concerned with the role that weight plays in the success of a knee or hip replacement that they often require their overweight patients to trim down before they'll even perform the operation. "Every extra pound that you carry magnifies what we call loading forces on the joint," says Dr. Laskowski. "That certainly puts more stress on the joint and the tissues around the joint."

Opt for an arch support. Not everyone who has flat feet has knee pain. But if you're of the flat-as-a-pancake persuasion and run a lot, you may get pain on the inner part of your knee. Orthotics for the arch of the foot, available either over the counter or from your doctor, help to correct an improper alignment of your leg that can cause knee pain, says Dr. Garry Sherman of Cedar Knolls, New Jersey. "I've had people who are a few days away from knee surgery come in. I make them orthotics, and their knee pain goes away," he says.

Backing into Fitness

Walking backward may seem like the worst possible way to get where you want to go. But if you have kneecap pain, there's evidence that walking backward will not only help you get better but also keep your cardiovascular system healthy while you rehabilitate.

Studies at William Beaumont Army Medical Center in El Paso, Texas, show that men who walked backward got a better workout than those walking forward at the same speed—even while reducing potentially damaging compression forces on the knee.

"This kills several birds with one stone," says Sean Connery, one of the lead authors of the studies and a clinical exercise physiologist in the center's Department of Clinical Investigation. "When you have knee pain, you get into this endless cycle: You can't exercise, you gain weight and that makes it worse on your knees when you try to exercise. But through backward running or backward walking you can strengthen the quadriceps muscles while staying fit—without kneecap pain."

Though these guys walked backward on treadmills, Connery suggests trying your reverse routine on a track for five minutes at a time, repeating four times and building from there.

Consider surgery. Unlike back surgery, studies show that knee operations are often successful. In the case of torn cartilage, the treatment consists of removing loose fragments and contouring the cartilage "so that it has a smooth edge that is less likely to get caught. It's not the best analogy, but it's like taking a nail clipper or file to a split fingernail so that it doesn't catch and turn into a big split," says Dr. Whipple.

Leg Pain

- Razor-sharp pain in your lower leg along the side of your shinbone

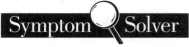

What It Means

You lace up your running shoes and hit the trail, a cedar-chip path snaking through oak and maple and walnut. A dove coos. Five miles today.

The crisp morning air pumps through your lungs like wind on a clean white sail. The sun, now orange against clear bright blue, breaks the horizon. In the back of your mind the Boss wails: "Tramps like us. . . baby we were born to ru-u-un. . . ." You reach the end and burst through the brush onto a country road, empty except for a kid on a bike carrying a sack bulging with newspapers. No. Ten today.

And it was bliss—every last step. But a day later you're hobbled with shin pain so bad that that jerk from marketing feels inclined to offer you a cane. What gives?

Though you had the best intentions, you fell victim to two of the most common causes of the leg pain commonly referred to as shinsplints: changing your running surface and logging too many miles.

You see, with every stride, there's a battle going on between your calf muscles and the muscles of your shin. "If your calf muscles aren't flexible, that puts more loading on the shins," says Bill Case, P.T., president of Case Physical Therapy in Houston. "The calf's job is to point your foot down. The muscles on the top of the leg—the shin muscles—pull your foot up. So if your calf muscles are tight and they are not allowing your shin muscles to pull up, the tug can create microtears in the muscles of the shin. Shinsplints."

All athletes—not just runners—are candidates for shinsplints. Run too long or on a surface that the muscles aren't used to and that

delicate balance between the calf and shin muscles has been upset—sometimes with painful results.

Symptom Solver

The real key to shinsplints is preventing them. Here are some tips to help you get over the ache and avoid a repeat performance.

Roll on the ice. Instead of laying an ice pack on your leg, freeze some water in a paper cup. Then peel down the sides for an ice massage on the sore area, says Dr. Darryl L. Kaelin of Outpatient Rehabilitation Services for Community Hospitals of Indianapolis. "If you rub the cup on your leg in a circular motion for 10 to 15 minutes after a workout, the ice goes right to work on the microtrauma and swelling," he says.

Stretch it out. There are lots of stretches that you can perform to avoid shinsplints, but one of the best goes like this: While seated with both feet flat on the floor in front of you, stretch the outside of one ankle by turning the bottom of that foot inward and pressing its outer side toward the ground. Hold for 15 to 30 seconds. Then turn the ankle so that the inside of the foot is pressing down toward the ground with the bottom of the foot turning outward. For both of these stretches, be sure to keep your knees up and out in front of your body in order to get the maximum stretch, says Dr. Kaelin. Repeat both stretches with the other ankle.

Here's another: While standing flat on one foot, place the toe of the other on the floor ahead and then rotate your ankle several times in a circle. Repeat in the opposite direction and repeat with the other foot.

Get stronger. Several sets of high-rep calf raises performed every other workout are also good for those with shinsplint pain, says Dr. Kaelin. With your shoes off, stand erect. Slowly rise onto your toes for a count of three. Lower and repeat 12 to 15 times. Dr. Kaelin suggests trying two or three sets with resting breaks between each set.

Wrap it. If you want to run through the injury, you'll probably need to cut back on mileage and intensity. You may also feel like you need some support. And we don't mean words of encouragement. Try using a 4-inch elastic bandage wrapped up the leg like a barber pole. Make sure that it's not too tight. You can wear it all day long but not while you sleep. Keep in mind, says Dr. Kaelin, that wrapping your leg in this manner won't heal your shinsplints, but it may be an additional help when exercising or stretching.

Get the right shoes. Big guys can't just slap on the same running shoes as their smaller brethren, crank out the mileage and expect to remain free of shinsplints, Case says. "If you're a big, heavy person that weighs 200 pounds or so and you're jogging in some flimsy shoe that you got at some discount store, it's like running barefoot," he warns. "By the same token, if you're a light person and you have a real hard shoe, you might as well be running in your street shoes."

For the most reliable and comprehensive information on all varieties of running shoes, check the spring or fall Shoe Buyer's Guide issues of *Runner's World* magazine, usually published each April and October. Or check the Runner's World Online shoe reviews on the World Wide Web at http://www.runnersworld.com.

Change shoes. You need to change your oil every 3,000 miles, right? Same principle with shoes. "You should change your running shoes every 300 to 350 miles—you just can't run forever in the same shoes. They lose their resiliency," Case says. If you aren't doing that much mileage but still run regularly, you might want to make a change every six months—or at least check to see how they're holding up.

Don't change sides. When running in the street, do you change sides on the way back? That could be contributing to your shinsplints. Because streets often slope to help water drain, you need to rebalance your body on the way back by running on the same side of the street, Case says.

Keep with softer surfaces. When possible, run on jogging tracks or grass—especially while recovering from shinsplints. If concrete is your only choice, remember to build up slowly, says Dr. Kaelin.

Shinsplint Prevention

Attach one end of a rope or some elastic exercise tubing to a low, anchored object like a dresser or a heavy chair and the other end to the ball of one foot. (Exercise tubing is more effective, but you will have to get it through your doctor or a physical therapist at a local rehabilitation center.)

While seated on a bed with one leg out in front of you and your foot fully extended, pull your foot and toes up toward your head for ten reps. Switch the rope or tubing to the other foot and repeat. Do three sets for each foot.

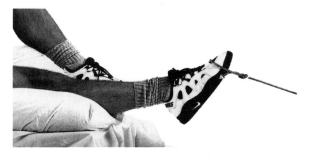

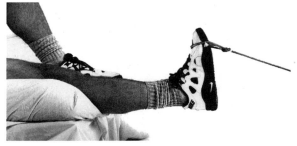

Muscle Cramps

- Your muscle seems locked in place

What It ❓ Means

There are times when you want to flex and show off your muscles—like in the bathroom after a shower when no one else is around.

And then there are times when one of your muscles decides that it wants to flex on its own. That painful involuntary muscle contraction is called a cramp.

You probably don't think about it, but what's really going on when you flex is that your muscle fibers contract and then expand. When you have a cramp, the muscle fibers contract—and freeze in that locked position. The result is incredibly painful and intense.

Two of the most common causes of cramps are lack of flexibility and dehydration. "Either you've worked the muscle all day and you didn't get it nice and flexible and stretched out afterward, or you've depleted your body of fluids and nutrients and haven't really replenished them. It's usually as simple as that," says Bill Case of Case Physical Therapy.

But it's not just while overexerting yourself that you can cramp up. It can happen while you sleep. Nocturnal leg cramps are a waking nightmare, which can be caused by a calf, hamstring or shin muscle getting locked in a contraction after a turn or stretch in your sleep.

Most experts recommend drinking six to eight glasses (eight ounces each) of water a day to keep cramps at bay, but if you're exercising or working in the heat, you're going to need much more. "In real hot weather, we give our athletes 24-ounce milkshake cups filled with water and ice every hour or so," says Morris Mellion, M.D., medical director of the Sports Medicine Center and clinical associate professor at the University of Nebraska Medical Center in Omaha.

If you want to know if you're losing too much water, you'll have to get naked. "The number one thing that you can do to prevent muscle cramps is to weigh yourself nude before and after exercise and make sure that you do not have a declining pattern of pre-exercise weight over a short period of time," Dr. Mellion says. "If you do, that's not from losing fat; that's from losing water. And that's when you get muscle cramps."

Symptom 🔍 Solver

When a muscle cramp kicks in, you want relief fast. Here's how to get it.

Slap on a lip lock. Although not all sports medicine experts are convinced, Michael Reed Gach, Ph.D., founder and director of the Acupressure Institute in Berkeley, California, and author of *Acupressure's Potent Points* says that squeezing the area between your nose and your lip activates an acupressure point that can quickly end a leg cramp. For best results, simply grab that fleshy part of your face between thumb and forefinger and squeeze until the cramp releases.

Stretch yourself. Whether it's in your calf, thigh or foot, nothing quite calms a muscle cramp like a slow, sustained stretch, says Case. Not only that, but elongated muscles are less likely to cramp in the future. Just remember: Never bounce when stretching, and hold the movement for 20 to 30 seconds for five reps.

Be kneaded. Deep massage at the heart of the cramped muscle performed either by yourself or by a friend may help relieve the cramp and restore normal motion, says Dr. Mellion.

Loosen up. If you occasionally suffer from nocturnal leg cramps, conduct a bed check. If your sheets and blankets are tight around your feet and lower legs, you may have your answer. Your leg gets caught in a mid-slumber turn and—ouch—you're suddenly awake and screaming. Try loosening the sheets before you turn in, says Case.

Neck Pain

• Your neck is stiff and sore

What It 🔍 Means

Piles of unpaid bills. In-laws. Car trouble. Add bona fide neck pain to these run-of-the-mill pains in the neck and you have problems, brother.

Of course, if your neck pain developed after a fall, car crash or some other accident, you should see your doctor. You may require medical treatment.

But chances are that you're just one of those guys who twists his neck muscles into awkward—and potentially painful—positions: watching television while lying down with your head and neck propped up, constantly holding a telephone receiver between your ear and shoulder or twisting to remove a pipe from a kitchen sink. Heck, even swinging a golf club can wrench your neck muscles to the point of pain.

If you're in pain, you don't have to take it lying down. In fact, a study of 300 back and neck pain sufferers found that self-treatment techniques such as exercise, heat and massage work better than painkillers and bed rest. "For muscular strain and overuse injuries like these, there's really nothing better," says Edward Hanley, M.D., chairman of the Department of Orthopaedics at Carolinas Medical Center in Charlotte, North Carolina.

Symptom 🔍 Solver

Experts recommend these tips to resolve your neck pain.

Have a ball. Place two tennis balls in the toes of a sock and knot the sock so that they don't move. Then lie down with your neck between the balls. The pressure should help the muscles in your neck relax.

Train a partner. A friend or partner can provide the same relief as the tennis ball treatment, only without the balls, simply by placing his fingers under your neck while you allow your head to relax and tilt back slightly.

Towel off. Fold a bath towel into thirds lengthwise. Grab one end with your left hand and one end with your right hand. Place the middle of the towel behind your head at the base of your skull. Let your head fall back, supported by the towel. Now pull the towel back and forth with your hands, allowing your head to be pulled with the towel. Breathe normally. You can do this for up to five minutes.

Massage with ice. An ice massage on the aching area will help reduce inflammation and pain. Freeze some water in a paper cup and then rub it on the injured area using a circular motion for 20 minutes every few hours for the first couple of days. "Ice has an analgesic effect and some muscle relaxant properties," says Dr. Hanley.

Turn up the heat. After a few days, switch to a heating pad or hot pack applied for 20 minutes a couple of times a day to help relax muscles and increase circulation, says Dr. Hanley.

Turn, turn, turn. Gently and carefully—but without in any way straining—try to turn your head from side to side. You may not be able to do much at first, but that's okay. Try again every hour or so. Slight movement can help a neck muscle in spasm to relax, experts say. (If you feel numbness, tingling or pain down your arm, stop immediately and see a doctor. These symptoms may be due to a pinched nerve, says Dr. Hanley.)

Consider a collar. For more severe pain, you may want to consider using a cervical neck collar, available at medical supply stores and some drugstores. It may provide temporary relief by immobilizing your neck, but if you wear one for more than a couple of days, it can weaken your neck muscles, says Dr. Hanley. And that can leave you more susceptible to further injury. So if your pain continues for more than three days, see your doctor.

Preventing Neck Pain

If you want to avoid future bouts, consider these tips.

Mind your posture. What seems like it would be a bigger strain on your neck: balancing the equivalent of a 16-pound bowling ball on top of your head or carrying it off to the side? Since your head roughly weighs as much as a large bowling ball, keep your head up straight. If you think you have posture problems, have a friend take a candid picture from the side. Then check it and see. "Your head is supposed to be positioned directly over your torso, which is directly situated over your pelvis and hips and heels. So if you do stand up straight, you're in balance, and you have to exert very little muscular effort to maintain that position," Dr. Hanley says.

See eye-to-eye with your computer. If you work at a computer, make sure that the middle of your monitor is just about eye level. "If you have to look down at the screen, then you're going to put excessive strain on your neck because your head is tilted forward," Dr. Hanley says.

Get a proper pillow. Instead of stacking up pillows pancake-style, use just one a few inches thick, preferably made from feathers. Too many pillows can stretch your neck muscles out of shape, Dr. Hanley says. But don't get one that's too soft and fluffy, he adds.

Take a break. Every hour or so, stand up from your chair and at least shrug your shoulders or turn your head gently from side to side. "You can't expect to sit there for three hours and not have tight muscles and pain," says Dr. Hanley.

Train those traps. The trapezius muscles—those triangle-shape jobs located on the upper back—are important for neck support. From now on when you visit the gym, pick up

Imagine . . .

What was it that the late John Lennon sang? *"Imagine there's no neck pain. It's easy if you try."* Well, maybe that wasn't it. But it could have been.

Dennis Gersten, M.D., a San Diego psychiatrist and publisher of *Atlantis*, a bimonthly imagery newsletter, says that you may be able to relieve neck pain by doing the following imagery exercise. He recommends doing it for ten minutes twice a day and whenever the pain flares up.

Picture your neck pain as a ball that has a particular size, shape, color and texture. It may be as small as a marble or as large as a basketball. Allow the ball to grow larger and larger. As it does, the pain may momentarily increase. Now let the ball shrink smaller than its original size, but don't let it disappear. As the intensity of the pain changes, allow the ball to change color, too. Now imagine that the ball turns into a liquid that flows down your arm, drips on the floor and reforms into a ball. Now kick or throw the ball out into space. Watch it disappear. Most of your pain should be gone.

a pair of 30-pound dumbbells and shrug your shoulders for three sets of 10 to 12 reps. "People with stronger neck muscles have fewer problems with chronic neck pain," says Dr. Hanley.

Practice necking in bed. Sorry, not that kind of necking. Lie on your bed on your stomach with your head hanging over the edge. Slowly lower your head as far as you comfortably can, then raise your head straight up and back (only up to 20 degrees past its straight level), bending only at the neck. Hold for a moment, then slowly lower your head again. Do two or three sets of 10 to 12 repetitions every other day to strengthen your neck muscles, says Dr. Hanley.

Shoulder Pain

- *You* need a shoulder to cry on

- You're unable to lift your arm over your head

- You have a dull ache in your shoulder

What It ❓ Means

Any shrewd businessman will tell you that there's an inverse relationship between overhead costs and profits. The same goes for overhead motion and shoulder health.

"Gymnastics, swimming, tennis—any overhead motion in and of itself, if done vigorously and repetitively, can cause damage to the shoulder," says Joseph Iannotti, M.D., Ph.D., associate professor of orthopedic surgery and chief of the shoulder and elbow service at the University of Pennsylvania in Philadelphia.

The main reason is that your shoulder's strong suit—wide range of motion—makes it that much easier to stress and strain tendons and ligaments. Unlike your hip joint, which has a deep ball-and-socket construction designed to maintain stability, your shoulder joint "has a small, shallow socket for a rather large ball—almost like a golf ball sitting on a golf tee," Dr. Iannotti says.

And without your rotator cuffs anchoring them in place, those big, broad shoulders of yours—the ones the gals love to cry on—wouldn't even support Kate Moss. "The rotator cuff is a mechanism that keeps the ball centered in the socket," says Dr. Iannotti. "As we learn more about shoulder biomechanics, it's hard not to have an appreciation of how important the rotator cuff is to maintaining shoulder stability."

It should come as no surprise, then, that rotator cuff tears, suffered by professional and weekend warriors alike, are one of the leading causes of shoulder pain, says Lanny L. Johnson, M.D., clinical professor in the Department of Surgery, College of Human Medicine, at Michigan State University in East Lansing.

What's more, some doctors believe that you can even damage your rotator cuff by sleeping with your arm over your head. "When you do this, you're pinching the rotator cuff tendon between the ball part of your upper arm bone and a prominent bone right on the top of the shoulder," Dr. Johnson says.

Land the wrong way playing flag football and you may dislocate your shoulder—literally pulling your arm bone out of your shoulder joint. Find yourself on the receiving end of a well-timed block during the same contest and you could separate your shoulder—a wrenching of the shoulder joint from the collarbone.

Painting a ceiling, hanging drywall and other overhead tasks can cause tendinitis, an irritation of tendons as they rub across bone. They also can cause bursitis, the swelling of fluid-filled sacs in your shoulder that normally help reduce friction.

Symptom 🔍 Solver

You don't have to suffer with prolonged shoulder pain. There are some obvious things that you can do, like taking aspirin, acetaminophen or any of the nonsteroidal anti-inflammatories available over the counter that help reduce swelling and provide temporary relief, says Dr. Johnson. And applying ice wrapped in a towel immediately after the pain flares helps soothe the ache and reduces swelling of inflamed tissues.

Each treatment session should last about 20 minutes, three times a day, says Dr. Iannotti. But here are some effective techniques that you may not have considered.

Sleep smart. Not every shoulder specialist believes that sleeping on your shoulder will cause pain, but those who do say that making an adjustment can avoid long-term damage. If you think how you sleep may be linked to your pain, try these positions: both arms at your side, bending one arm at the elbow and placing the pillow between the palm of your hand and your head, and placing your pillow between your elbow, forearm and your head, says Dr. Johnson.

Get limber. While waiting for your shoulder to recover, try this exercise: With your good arm against a desk for support, bend at the waist and let your affected arm hang down to the floor. Now gently swing your arm back and forth like a slow pendulum. "This allows the shoulder to limber up without putting any stress on the tendons or muscles," says Dr. Johnson.

Let gravity help. Here's another helpful exercise: Lie on your back, straighten your arms out at your side and lift your hands until your arms are over your head. Slowly allow your arms and hands to touch the floor above your head. "This is a way to gain full elevation of your arm with a minimal load to tendons and muscles—gravity assists you in gaining the elevation," Dr. Johnson says. "If you were standing up, you'd have to be lifting your arm up against gravity."

Go for a clean sweep. Holding a broomstick behind your back with your palms up, slowly raise your hands as far as possible away from you. Hold for a two count. Slowly lower and repeat ten times, says Dr. Iannotti.

Identify, then modify. The logic behind this tip is at the heart of one of the oldest doctor jokes in the world. (Patient: "Doc, it hurts when I do this." Doc: "So don't do it.") But by changing the movement that's causing your shoulder pain, you may be able to avoid it altogether, says Joseph Askinasi, a chiropractic orthopedist in New York City. "If you're able to link your ache to your killer tennis serve, you may not have to give up tennis, but you should probably change your serve."

Turn on the heat. Dull, persistent shoulder pain may improve with a daily application of the hot stuff. For no more than 20 minutes at a time, apply a heating pad or a damp washcloth warmed in the microwave. (The cloth should be warm to the touch but not

so hot that it will burn your skin.) "Heat helps increase blood flow to the area and helps loosen some of the tissues. It's particularly good for someone suffering from bursitis or tendinitis," says Dr. Iannotti. Some athletes even apply heat before exercising to help prepare their shoulders for a workout.

Lay low. For moderate shoulder pain, avoid your regular shoulder exercise for three to four weeks. Avoid reaching, lifting, pushing or pulling activities above the waist, says Dr. Iannotti. More serious injuries may need six weeks or more to heal.

"If you don't take off enough time to resolve the problem, you'll think that you have a chronic problem. But you don't. You're just converting a minor problem to a chronic problem," says Dr. Johnson.

Minimize your military presses. In your quest for bolder shoulders, are you trying to max out your military presses? This could be the source of your pain and long-term damage to your rotator cuff, says Dan O'Neill, M.D., medical director of the St. John Sports Medicine Center in Nassau Bay, Texas. Instead, never perform military presses with more than 60 percent of your one-rep max. "You don't have to abandon the exercise altogether—just keep it light and go for higher repetitions," he says.

Warm up. If you're going to pump iron, warm up by doing lateral raises and upright rows with one- to two-pound dumbbells for a few minutes before starting the more strenuous part of your workout.

Get thee to a PT. If self-treatments don't seem to help and your doctor is talking surgery, consider seeing a physical therapist. In a British study that compared the results of shoulder surgery, exercise and a placebo or blank pill, researchers found that those folks who participated in a supervised exercise program for six months did as well as those who went under the knife. Instead of carving out room for inflamed tendons through surgery, the right exercise can help strengthen the muscles and tendons of the rotator cuff.

Wrist Pain

- Wrist pain or numbness radiates up your arm or through your hand and fingers

What It ❓ Means

Which is worse? You be the judge.
- Lincoln Tunnel syndrome: Stuck in bumper-to-bumper, rush-hour traffic hell in an exhaust-filled, underwater tube heading into New York City
- Carpal tunnel syndrome: Stuck at a computer terminal for hours on end with pain and numbness shooting from your fingertips to your shoulder

Tough call. But if you've ever suffered from carpal tunnel syndrome, you'd probably be happy to take your chances in the Lincoln Tunnel.

Yes, it's that painful.

A narrow passage inside your wrist, your carpal tunnel is home to nine tendons and your median nerve—all encased in a slippery sheath called the synovium. When the synovium and tendons become inflamed and swollen, they squeeze the median nerve.

Pressure from the pinched median nerve sends a typically dull pain, numbness and tingling radiating through your hand and two or three fingers and an accompanying ache in your forearm. Sometimes the pain is so intense that it can wake you from a sound sleep.

Although women suffer from carpal tunnel syndrome more often than men, there are certain guys who are prime candidates, says Dr. Terry Whipple of the University of Virginia School of Medicine.

What kind of men? "Those with thick connective tissues: dense skin on their palms; less flexible joints; broad, thick hands; heavy jawbones—basically thicker tissues—that sort of body build," says Dr. Whipple. As these tissues age, he says, they actually become more dense and less flexible, crowding the nerve and causing pain.

But it's not just thick-skinned computer jockeys who risk the painful problem. Occupations requiring a power grip also are likely causes. "Men who use tin snips in the sheet metal shop, swing a hammer, carve meat at the butcher shop, even doing long-distance cycling in that awkward racing position—those kinds of things can strain tendons. And as they swell, they crowd the nerve," says Dr. Whipple. Debate still rages whether repetitive activity such as typing or assembly work causes carpal tunnel syndrome.

And as if you really needed another reason to kick the butts, smoking can contribute to the onset of carpal tunnel syndrome, he says. "Smoking alters your peripheral circulation, and by altering your peripheral circulation, it can damage the health of the nerves," Dr. Whipple says.

Wrist Risks

Diabetes can actually mimic the wrist pain symptoms of carpal tunnel syndrome. "It's very similar. You lose keen sensation and develop weakness of grip strength," says Dr. Whipple.

High blood pressure and kidney dysfunction, too, can cause increased fluid retention, which is one of the most common causes of the problem in women.

Falling on your outstretched hand and spraining your wrist—an obvious cause of wrist pain—may also contribute to carpal tunnel syndrome. "If your wrist swells as a result, that swelling can compress the nerve," says Dr. Whipple. But such a fall is more likely to actually break your wrist. (If you still have pain a week after such a fall, see your doctor—you may have fractured your wrist.)

Even repeatedly gripping and swinging a

tennis racket, baseball bat or golf club can stress the tendons and ligaments of the wrist, causing swelling, pain, numbness or tingling.

While living with the pain may seem like the easiest thing to do, you could be setting yourself up for some long-term problems, warns J. Lee Berger, M.D., assistant clinical professor of orthopedics at Seton Hall Graduate School of Medicine in South Orange, New Jersey. "If you wait too long and you do have carpal tunnel syndrome, you can cause irreversible damage," Dr. Berger says.

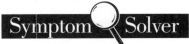

Ready to put your wrist pain to rest? You probably know that if you've recently taken a dive on your outstretched wrist, your first course of action should be to ice it. Place an ice pack or water frozen in a paper cup on your wrist for 15 to 20 minutes several times a day, says Dr. Berger. This will help reduce swelling and ease the ache. Here are some other proven methods of easing the pain.

Beat it while you sleep. Men who snooze in a fetal position with their hands under their heads, or on their stomachs with their arms curled under their chest seem to be at a greater risk for night pain caused by carpal tunnel syndrome, says Dr. Whipple.

"These positions narrow the space through which the nerve passes. That's what wakes you up in the middle of the night with this tingling and dead feeling in your fingers," he says. To avoid the pain, try training yourself to sleep on your back with your hands at your side.

Spring for some splints. If you can't seem to get the hang of a new sleeping style on your own, check into some wrist splints. Worn at night, they help prevent you from flexing your wrists while you sleep. "That might be all that you need to control the symptoms until your tendons have the chance to shrink back to size," says Dr. Whipple. Although splints are appropriate for certain causes of carpal tunnel syndrome, not everyone will benefit, he says. Available in drugstores, night splints cost about $20.

Boost your vitamin B$_6$. Since carpal tunnel syndrome is linked to the swelling of tissues, what could work better than a natural

Wrist Stretches

Raise your left arm as if you are commanding traffic to stop. Place your right hand over your left palm and gently pull your left hand back. Repeat with your opposite arm and hand.

With your left arm out and your left fingers pointing down, place your right hand over your left hand and gently pull. Repeat with your opposite arm and hand. Consider performing these when you take a break every hour or so.

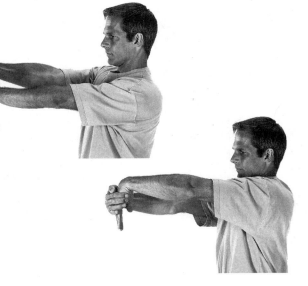

diuretic like vitamin B$_6$? "It pulls fluid out of tissues and dumps it from the body through the kidneys," says Dr. Whipple. "By pulling fluid from the tissues, it reduces some of the swelling adjacent to the nerve. So if you have a temporary condition in which the nerve has become crowded, vitamin B$_6$ may help.

You'll need to take 300 milligrams of vitamin B$_6$ a day for up to 12 weeks for the best result, he says. But be aware: Research shows that high doses of vitamin B$_6$ can be toxic, and unstable gait and numb feet may occur in doses of B$_6$ at 50 milligrams to 2 grams daily over a prolonged time. The Daily Value for vitamin B$_6$ is 2 milligrams. A single serving of foods high in vitamin B$_6$—potatoes, bananas and chickpeas—doesn't even provide a single milligram of B$_6$.

Stretch yourself. Could hand and wrist stretches help eliminate wrist pain in those with occupational injuries? That's the possibility raised by at least one university study. Researchers found that when 28 people learned and practiced a yoga-based regimen of exercises twice a week for ten weeks (for an hour each time), they had less pain than 27 others who wore wrist splints.

Go in reverse. Regular and reverse wrist curls can strengthen your arm muscles and help you avoid sports-related wrist pain, experts say. For regular wrist curls, simply hold a light dumbbell palm up in one hand over the edge of a bench or table. Without lifting your wrist off the surface, slowly curl the weight up ten times. Repeat with the other wrist.

To perform reverse wrist curls, hold the weight palm down and repeat as above. Experts suggest three sets of ten lifts, once or twice a day.

Floating a Trial Balloon

If the thought of surgery for your carpal tunnel syndrome makes you cringe, there's good news on the horizon. A New Jersey doctor has developed a surgical technique that seems to relieve chronic carpal tunnel pain with less reliance on the knife.

Called balloon carpal tunnel-plasty, the procedure helps ease the pain the same way that some cardiac specialists unclog arteries of the heart, says Dr. J. Lee Berger of Seton Hall Graduate School of Medicine.

In layman's terms, a balloon-type device is inserted in the carpal tunnel and then is expanded, widening the pathway and relieving pressure on the nerve, Dr. Berger says.

"Carpal tunnel syndrome is what we call a compressive neuropathy—where you have a ligament that presses on the nerve. I thought that if I could come up with a way that takes the pressure off the nerve without cutting the ligament, it would solve a lot of problems," says Dr. Berger. Although relatively safe and effective, the traditional method of cutting wrist ligaments during carpal tunnel surgery has been linked to weakened grip strength in patients and requires several weeks of recovery.

After several years of developing the equipment and refining the technique, Dr. Berger began performing his operation. A four-year, nine-month follow-up shows that among 130 patients, his technique has a 92 percent success rate.

"Most people who have the traditional procedure are out of work for four to six weeks. It took our patients about ten days before they were ready to return to work," says Dr. Berger, who is seeking Food and Drug Administration approval of the equipment needed for the procedure.

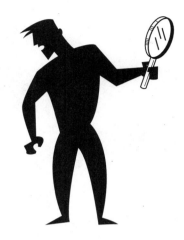

Part Seven

Skin

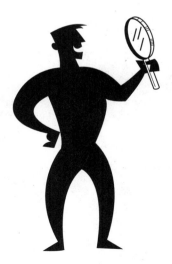

Acne

- You chaperone the junior high dance—and the kids make fun of your face

- You get occasional pimples

What It Means

As you suffered with pimples in your teen years, you could draw some small solace from the fact that almost everyone else your age was going through the same thing. But the only real consolation lay in the sure knowledge that it was something that you would eventually grow out of.

Now your twenty-fifth high school reunion is looming on the horizon, and you're still wondering when you'll outgrow acne. In fact, you're as worried about pimples as you were before the prom. What kind of cruel joke is this?

The problem goes back to puberty. That's when your hormones trigger glands mostly located on your face, chest and upper back to start producing large amounts of an oily substance called sebum, which lubricates the skin.

For 80 percent of us, that's when pimples begin. The sebum sometimes spills into the skin, plugging up oil glands, which eventually swell, turn red and fill with pus. Sebum also can cause pimples by feeding bacteria lurking in the skin.

As you get older, sebum levels drop—but they don't disappear.

"It's a myth that it stops once you turn 20. It slows down, but it doesn't stop," says Mitchell C. Stickler, M.D., a dermatologist in private practice in Lewes, Delaware. "They never really stop. Even elderly people will get whiteheads under the skin, though the pimples usually aren't as inflamed as they were during puberty."

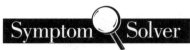

Whether you have bad acne is largely a matter of genetics. It doesn't have much to do with your personal hygiene. Dirt doesn't cause pimples. Oil does. That's why scrubbing your skin won't clear up pimples. It might actually irritate them. "I recommend that my patients do not use washcloths or polyester scrub sponges. You should just wash gently with your fingertips and lightly pat dry with a soft towel when done," says Nelson Lee Novick, M.D., associate clinical professor of dermatology at Mount Sinai School of Medicine in New York City. Stick to gently washing your face only two times a day with a mild, nonsoap cleanser such as Cetaphil lotion.

And use the following tips to create a clearer complexion.

Buy benzoyl peroxide. Despite advertising claims, over-the-counter acne products don't zap existing zits into oblivion. But they do help prevent pimples by either halting bacterial growth or opening pores. "You have to use them daily. They don't do much once you have a pimple," warns Dr. Stickler.

What you buy over the counter will contain either benzoyl peroxide or salicylic acid. The benzoyl peroxide gels such as Johnson and Johnson's Clean & Clear work best, especially on oily skin, Dr. Stickler says. For those with dry, sensitive skin, lotions and creams are less irritating.

Put egg on your face. To make a pimple go poof, crack an egg and get some of the egg white on a cotton swab and apply it to the blemish. "Egg white is a mild astringent—meaning that it can help tighten the skin—and probably contains some anti-inflammatory proteins," says James Fulton, M.D., a dermatologist in private practice in Newport Beach, California.

Peel it. Alpha hydroxy acids won their fame because they reduce wrinkles. But they have another plus. The constant exfoliation keeps the pores clean, Dr. Stickler says. Various over-the-counter moisturizers contain alpha hydroxy acids up to 10 percent. You can get a stronger cream by prescription from your dermatologist.

Eat right. Foods don't cause acne. But certain foods can make it worse in some people. They include chocolate, nuts, carbonated beverages and milk, says Dr. Stickler. Also, the grease from fast foods usually won't cause acne—unless you get it on your skin. So wash up after you eat french fries or other greasy treats.

Use clean moisture. When buying moisturizers, make sure they are noncomedogenic, says Dr. Stickler. That means that they won't cause pimples.

Keep your hands off. If you habitually lean your face on your palm, you'll clog your pores and develop pimples. Dr. Stickler often sees teenagers with pimples around the area of their football helmet strap.

Don't obsess. "You don't have to examine your skin with a magnifying glass in search of a possible blemish," says Tabitha Henderson, M.D., senior director of dermatology research for Ortho Pharmaceutical in Raritan, New Jersey. People who look too closely can end up picking and gouging their skin, which can lead to more blemishes and possible scarring.

Get it opened. There's a way to pop a pimple that will make it go away faster. But you shouldn't do it yourself. A doctor can use a needle to open your pores for you. But it must be done carefully with a sterile needle. "It's best if a professional opens them," Dr. Stickler says. If you pick at your pimples, you'll likely get them infected or create scarring.

Enlist a professional. Your dermatologist can prescribe a number of methods to clear up stubborn acne cases, Dr. Stickler says. One is to use prescription tretinoin (Retin-A)

Dial "A" for Acne

If you think telemarketers are annoying, well, you're right. But they may not be the *most* annoying thing about your telephone.

That dubious distinction may belong to a phenomenon known as "phone acne." If you spend a lot of time each day working the phones, and you have acne flaring up on your chin, there may be a connection. When you rest the phone against your chin, it can activate acne there. The mouthpiece presses against hair follicles, blocking facial oils.

And it's not just the phone that can reach out and touch off acne. Resting your chin in your hand while you're reading or wearing a headband when you're working out can also block follicles.

What can you do? "Keep your phone receiver clean with alcohol and teach yourself to hold the phone just a centimeter away from your face," says Anita Cela, M.D., clinical asssistant professor of dermatology at Cornell University Medical College in New York City.

Using a headset is another way to avoid the problem. And it has the added benefit of relieving potential neck problems as well.

with regular glycolic acid peels. The two creams remove material from your skin that can block pores. Each acid peel will leave your face red and irritated for a few days. For really severe acne, you can take isotretinoin (Accutane), a powerful prescription drug that usually keeps skin acne-free for a year or longer by reducing the amount of oil in the skin. Accutane has a number of side effects, ranging from chapped lips to joint pain to liver problems.

Athlete's Foot and Jock Itch

- Your feet are itchy
- Your feet are peeling
- Your groin is itchy
- The skin around your groin is red and scaly

What It Means

A baseball player saunters slowly up to the plate, grabs his groin and whacks the bat against his cleat. *We* think that he's loosening up and refining his stance. *He's* thinking: "Ahhh. Got it."

It's not the kind of statistic that you'll find on trading cards, but athletes are prime candidates for jock itch and athlete's foot, both caused by fungi that thrive in moist, warm environments—like between the toes and in the groin area.

You don't have to whack balls around for a living to experience the fierce itching, peeling and redness of either of these conditions. You can pick up a fungus in any damp environment, like a locker room, steam room, swimming pool or even your own bathroom. In fact, the fungi are everywhere, although some people are more susceptible to infection than others. In addition, you can be infected without having symptoms—at least until the itching flares.

Itchy skin isn't always caused by athlete's foot. Some people have eczema, an itchy rash often caused by dry skin, says K. William Kitzmiller, M.D., volunteer clinical professor of dermatology at the University of Cincinnati and spokesman for the American Academy of Dermatology.

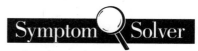
Symptom Solver

Jock itch tends to cause a "damp" rash in the groin area. Athlete's foot can be either a damp or dry rash on the soles of the feet. Try lubricating dry rashes with a hydrating cream such as Nivea lotion and use a mild soap like Dove, says Dr. Kitzmiller.

But if you suspect that you have athlete's foot or jock itch, try these remedies.

Kill the fungus. You don't need us to tell you to throw some antifungal ointment in the cart the next time you're at the grocery store. But you may need some help picking the right kind. A study from the Cleveland Veterans Affairs Medical Center found that over-the-counter products containing miconazole (like Monistat 7) are the most cost-effective. Look for a store-brand generic that uses miconazole as the active ingredient.

Apply the ointment to the skin twice a day, says Dr. Mitchell C. Stickler of Lewes, Delaware. Make sure to use the medicine for a few weeks after the infection clears up.

If over-the-counter products don't help, your doctor may recommend an antifungal medication taken orally, says Dr. Stickler.

Make your own. Mix two teaspoons of table salt per pint of warm water and then soak your feet for 5 to 15 minutes at a time. "The salt kills fungus and helps to dry up surface skin cells," says Glenn Copeland, D.P.M., podiatrist for the Toronto Blue Jays professional baseball team and author of *The Foot Doctor*. You can also try soaking for 10 to 15 minutes in a solution made with a half-cup of white vinegar in a gallon of warm water, he says.

But beware: Do-it-yourself concoctions are not nearly as strong as the antifungal agents that you can buy at the store. They may keep the fungus in check, but they probably won't cure the problem, cautions Dr. Stickler.

Stay dry. The fungus likes moisture. So you can prevent further outbreaks by not feeding it fluids. According to Dr. Stickler, here are some basic strategies.

- Don't overlook your toes. Make sure that you dry yourself thoroughly after a shower to eliminate the wet environment that the fungus loves. Be sure to include the area between the toes.
- Wear loose cotton underwear and cotton socks. Some synthetics such as Coolmax also are a good choice because they pull moisture away from the skin. But avoid older synthetics such as polyester because they hold water against your skin.
- Apply baby powder without cornstarch once or twice a day.
- Alternate between two or three pairs of shoes so that they have a chance to dry between wears. This will also make your shoes last longer because dampness is what breaks down the leather.
- Wash gym clothes, underwear and athletic supporters between wearings.
- If your feet sweat a lot, apply antiperspirant. You should use separate antiperspirants for feet and underarms to prevent possible spread of fungus.

Use garlic. Raw garlic has natural antifungal properties. "Put chopped garlic in your socks before bedtime and then wear them overnight," says Julian Whitaker, M.D., founder and president of the Whitaker Wellness Center in Newport Beach, California.

Practice prevention. The best way to prevent athlete's foot or jock itch is to prevent the fungus from getting to your skin. So wear rubber flip-flops whenever you are showering away from home, says Tobias Samo, M.D., clinical associate professor at Baylor College of Medicine in Houston. Also, use your own

---

Trail Mix

Perhaps the only good thing that you can say about athlete's foot is that it leaves your hands free to scratch. But imagine that you're a deer and you have athlete's hoof (yes, they do get it).

You don't have hands to scratch with. There aren't stores in the forest that sell antifungal ointments. Even if there were, how would you spread it on your hooves? With your antlers?

As it turns out, deer may have a built-in plan for combating athlete's hoof. Until recently, scientists thought that glands in deer's hooves were used to leave scents behind for other deer. But William Wood, Ph.D., professor of chemistry at Humboldt State University in Arcata, California, has found that the substance, a simple ketone, has antibacterial and antifungal properties. He doesn't know for sure, but he guesses that it helps deer combat the athlete's foot (or hoof) fungus.

Deer ailments aside, the discovery could help people overcome a range of bacterial and fungal ailments, from athlete's foot and acne to dandruff. Now that he knows what the substance is, Dr. Wood says that he can make it synthetically. So deer don't need to line up and volunteer their glands for the sake of human athlete's foot.

---

towel, not one from the gym.

Athlete's foot can spread from your feet to your groin. So dry off from top to bottom, not vice versa. And put your socks on before putting on your underwear. Otherwise you might drag the fungus upward, says Keith Schulze, M.D., a dermatologist in private practice in Wharton, Texas.

Body Odor

• When you untie your shoelaces, your kids pull their shirts over their faces

• Someone at work keeps putting soap and deodorant in your desk drawer

What It Means

In high school, an unlaundered gym uniform was more than a badge of honor. It was a potent good luck charm.

A team could win or lose, depending on how spoiled it smelled. At least that's what everyone thought.

"When I was in high school, we used to wash our gym uniforms maybe once every two weeks. There was a joke about the smellier your uniform was, the more of a man you were," says Tom Easton, senior director of product development for The Body Shop, an international manufacturer and retailer of skin, hair and cosmetic products. "But the days when a smelly pair of sweatpants or sweatsocks were appealing to anybody are way over with."

Of course, there's more to body odor than washing your gym clothes—or yourself. Everyone has his own personal smell. Some people are sweeter than others. Some are fouler. Some are mild. And some are strong.

Strong body smells generally come from a by-product of sweat—more specifically, from the type of sweat produced by glands (the apocrine glands) most prominent in the armpits and groin. These glands secrete a milky substance that bacteria love. The sweat clings to underarm and pubic hair, allowing bacteria to have a field day. As the sweat breaks down, it begins to smell. The kind of smell depends on the makeup of your apocrine sweat. And that's determined by genetics, age, sex, race, culture and ethnicity.

Hormones control your apocrine glands.

That's why body odors aren't a problem until you hit puberty. As you age, the reverse happens; you'll begin to smell less as hormone levels gradually decline.

Unlike sweat from the apocrine glands, that produced by the eccrine glands—the salty, colorless fluid that appears when you exercise—is rarely odoriferous. But when you eat strong foods like garlic or onions, you can sometimes smell them in the eccrine sweat.

A condition called hyperhidrosis, or excessive sweating, can intensify body odor. In such people, the underarms and other body parts such as the palms and feet can produce huge amounts of sweat, meaning more food for bacteria. "There are some people who have really bad sweating of the palms. They can't shake hands. You can often see wet marks on their pants from where they've wiped their hands," says Dr. Mitchell C. Stickler of Lewes, Delaware.

Before you go about trying to eliminate smells from your body, keep in mind that body odor does serve a function. Scientists have known for some time that animals use one another's distinctive body odors in mating. And they've uncovered evidence that humans do much the same thing.

Researchers in Switzerland asked women to sniff various T-shirts that had been worn by deodorantless men for two nights. The women were asked to rank the smells as either pleasant or unpleasant. The researchers found that women were attracted to the smells of men who had different genetic makeups than their own. And that makes sense. Mating with someone whose DNA is different than your own gives your offspring a better chance of survival.

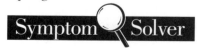

Symptom Solver

Sweat doesn't smell unless it gets trapped. And your feet and armpits are prime regions for trapped sweat. (If you wore gloves all day, eventually your hands would smell, too, says Dr. Stickler.) To treat body odor, you basically have three strategies. You can decrease the amount of sweat. You can make sure that the sweat gets off your body pronto. Or you can use other smells to mask your own smell. Here are some things that you may want to try.

Make friends with your shoes. You need at least three pairs of shoes, says Dr. Stickler. The idea is to have enough shoes that you never wear the same pair two days in a row. You want to allow them to dry out between wearings, says Dr. Stickler. Not only will this cut down on foot odor; it also helps shoes last longer, he adds.

Kill the bacteria. Using an antibacterial soap such as Lever 2000, Dial or Safeguard will help keep body odors at manageable levels, says Dr. Stickler.

Ban the smell. There are three types of products that can help quell underarm smell. There's deodorant. There's antiperspirant. There's deodorant-antiperspirant combinations. You definitely want at least an antiperspirant, if not a combo, since this blocks or cuts down on the amount of sweat that eventually creates the smell in the first place. All that a plain deodorant does is mask the odor with perfume, Dr. Stickler says.

Don't leave out your feet. The same thing that stops sweating in your armpits can stop it on your feet. So don't forget to slide the antiperspirant on your soles if excessive sweating is a problem, says Dr. Stickler. You should use separate antiperspirants on your feet and underarms to prevent the possible spread of fungus.

Have dry dreams. Antiperspirants work best if you apply them the night before you need them to work, says Dr. Stickler. If you have an especially bad problem, apply antiperspirants to the palms and feet, and cover them up with disposable gloves for the night, Dr. Stickler says. Or use plastic bags held in place with socks.

Let yourself breathe. Stay away from clothing that doesn't "breathe," such as

polyester. First, it will make you hotter, and you'll sweat more. Second, it'll trap sweat, creating a bacteria feeding frenzy. For breathability, the best fabric is cotton, says Dr. Stickler.

Get stronger treatment. If you have severe sweating, over-the-counter antiperspirants may not help. You can get a stronger prescription antiperspirant—containing 20 percent aluminum chloride hexahydrate alcoholic solution (Drysol)—from a dermatologist, says Dr. K. William Kitzmiller of the University of Cincinnati.

Stop Making Scents

Using too much scent doesn't make sense; it's just one of many fragrance faux pas that men unwittingly commit every day. Even the most well-groomed of us can use a few pointers in the artificial smell department. So we called Tom Easton of The Body Shop and asked him to set us in the right direction. Here's his advice.

1. Avoid the "potpourri effect." This happens when you shower with Safeguard, roll Old Spice under your arms, splash on a minty aftershave and top it off with a sweet-smelling hair spray. "You don't want 17 different smells going on. All that you'll do is end up attracting bees," says Easton. What you want to do is "layer" your fragrances—buy a shampoo, aftershave, deodorant and soap that have similar smells.

2. Don't jump in the bottle. Some products are very strong because they contain a lot of oil. That's why they are also expensive. You don't want to put such products directly on your skin or you'll end up leaving a trail of cologne everywhere you go. Instead, put a little spritz in the air, then walk into the mist.

3. Pick the right smell. Skin reacts to fragrances in different ways. That's why it's not a good idea to let your girlfriend choose your cologne unless you try it on first. When purchasing cologne, spray a sample on your skin. Then walk around for a while to let the fragrance interact with you. Wait about 20 minutes. Then decide whether you like the smell.

Bruises

- A bluish-purple mark on your skin

What It Means

Bruises usually mean one of two things: Something mobile—your body—traveled into something immobile—a wall. Or something mobile—someone's fist—traveled into something mobile—your face.

There are, of course, endless combinations. But the result is always the same: The contact makes blood vessels just beneath the skin's surface break and bleed. And when that happens, it's good to have thick skin. It's the blood showing through the skin that gives us that black-and-blue look. The thinner the skin, the more noticeable the bruise.

Bruises usually start out a bluish-purple color. Later, as parts of the blood break down, the bruise turns yellowish-green and then brown.

As you age, you'll bruise more easily, especially on the backs of your arms, says Dr. Mitchell C. Stickler of Lewes, Delaware. That's because years of sun exposure make the walls of the blood vessels thin, leaving them more fragile, he says.

Symptom Solver

The best thing to do is not get them. That means protecting your body by wearing padding while playing football, in-line skating and while performing other activities, says Dr. K. William Kitzmiller of the University of Cincinnati.

But you can't always move throughout the world with a protective body shield. So here are a few ways to thwart those ugly black-and-blue marks.

Try special K. Vitamin K cream will make a bruise go away faster, Dr. Stickler says.

Vitamin K is a blood clot regulator that's commonly given to patients orally before plastic surgery to reduce bruising. Researchers found that it can reduce bruising through the skin as well. But they aren't sure why it works. (Don't assume that oral vitamin K is a substitute for the cream form. In fact, it can be harmful.)

Slap on a steak. Every cowboy—and everyone who grew up watching old westerns—knows what a man's gotta do after a rip-roarin', knock-down, drag-out barroom brawl. You saunter on over to the chuck wagon, grab a slab of raw beef and slap it on your black eye. It turns out that those old cowpokes may have been right. Steak is high in vitamin K, which may speed recovery from bruising, Dr. Stickler says. It's also cold, so it will reduce swelling.

You booze, you bruise. If you're going to be in a barroom brawl, the last thing that you want to do is drink alcohol. Of course, if you're not drinking alcohol, your odds of getting into a barroom brawl seem pretty slim. But that's beside the point. Booze makes you bruise more easily because it thins your blood, making it easier to leak into the skin, says Dr. Stickler. The same goes for aspirin. If you need to kill the pain of getting whacked in the eye, take acetaminophen.

Put a plant on it. No, not a potted poinsettia. That's too heavy. It'll probably give you another bruise. Try a gel derived from the arnica plant. "Arnica is soothing and has a local anti-inflammatory effect that can speed healing," says George Fareed, M.D., who specializes in sports medicine at Pioneers Medical Center in Brawley, California. Apply the gel two to four times a day. It will make the bruise fade within four days, much less time than if you just grin and bear it. You can buy the gel at health food stores.

Cover your skin. When you're out in the sun, smear on some sunscreen with a sun protection factor (SPF) of at least 15. That will help prevent the age-related increase in bruising, Dr. Stickler says.

Cold Sores

- Lip sore that blisters then scabs

- Lip sore sometimes preceded by itching and burning

What It 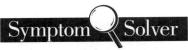 Means

First, the bad news: You have herpes.

Now, the good news: It's possible, if this is your first cold sore, that you'll never get one again.

But don't count on it. Once you're infected with the cold sore–causing herpesvirus, you never really get rid of it. Even when the sores are gone from your skin, the virus is safe and secure deep within your nerves.

Chances are that the sores eventually will pop up again at various times, especially when you are under stress, out in the sun or are sick.

There are two types of herpesviruses that can cause cold sores. Type 1 causes 60 percent of the cold sores on the lips and face, with the rest being caused by the Type 2 virus, which tends to be more severe. On the genitals, the percentages of the two types are reversed, with Type 2 predominating.

The virus is very contagious. Even when you don't have a cold sore, you can spread it. "Someone who doesn't even know that he has herpes can give someone else a really severe case of it," says Dr. Mitchell C. Stickler of Lewes, Delaware.

The virus is most contagious, however, when you have a blistering sore, says Dr. Stickler. It can spread from your lips to someone else's—or from your lips to their genitals.

And you don't need direct contact. You can spread the virus by using the same linens, towels or toothbrushes.

A cold sore usually starts out with an itching, burning and tingling feeling. Then a red sore forms. It blisters. Then the blister breaks open, and a scab forms.

The whole scenario takes about two weeks.

Symptom Solver

Cold sores are very difficult to avoid. Ninety percent of the population has either a Type 1 or Type 2 virus, says Dr. K. William Kitzmiller of the University of Cincinnati. Avoiding close contact with people who have cold sores and not using someone else's towels and linens are some of the best ways to avoid them. When you do get them, here are a few ways to shorten their duration.

Get a prescription. Taking the prescription medication acyclovir (Zovirax) has been shown to shorten cold-sore outbreaks by about half, to as little as seven days. Acyclovir is sold in oral and topical forms. You have to take it orally to get good results, Dr. Stickler says. The cream form will only shorten the duration of a cold sore by about a day.

Keep it clean. When you have a sore, wash the area twice a day with Dove, Basis or another mild soap to prevent infection. Applying an over-the-counter antibacterial ointment like Polysporin to the area once or twice a day will also help prevent infection, says Dr. Stickler.

Keep it home. Herpes is transmitted by kissing and other types of close contact. And don't share towels or linens with someone who is currently in the midst of an outbreak, Dr. Stickler says.

Keep it locked up. To prevent the herpesvirus from coming out of hiding, try to avoid stress and excessive sunlight, two of the most common cold-sore triggers. You can avoid outbreaks by wearing sunscreen and lowering your stress levels, says Dr. Stickler. Exercise, eat a balanced diet and make sure to get between six and eight hours of sleep.

Dandruff

- Your scalp is itchy, flaky and red

What It Means

Every 24 days you shed your skin.

You may be thinking, "I have never shimmied out of a layer of skin, leaving a gossamery likeness of myself behind." And you're right. Humans don't shed skin the way that snakes do. But our skin cells do shed. They just do it at different times. This happens all over our bodies, but the only place we usually notice it is on the head or eyebrows, where hairs catch the flakes, says Dr. Mitchell C. Stickler of Lewes, Delaware. The resulting flakes are generally known as dandruff.

A flaky scalp isn't always caused by skin shedding off. Excess oiliness can create greases and fatty acids that cause dryness, redness, scaling, itching and irritation says Dr. K. William Kitzmiller of the University of Cincinnati.

Yeasts commonly found on the skin can inflame the scalp, causing a scaly, red rash. This condition, called seborrheic dermatitis, can also affect other body parts, such as the eyebrows. It's an inherited condition that occurs more frequently as people age, Dr. Stickler says.

Also, a skin condition called psoriasis can make skin cells grow faster than normal and form red scaly patches. It is not contagious, but it is itchy and annoying.

Symptom Solver

Daily shampooing takes care of the normal flakes caught in your hair. You only need to use a mild, nonmedicated shampoo, says Dr. Stickler. But for more severe dandruff, you'll need stronger treatment. Here's what to do.

Set it free. Wearing a tight hat can make dandruff worse, as can the heavy use of hair sprays and gels, says Dr. Stickler.

What's more, hair products can produce their own flakes that resemble dandruff, says Dr. Nelson Lee Novick of Mount Sinai School of Medicine. Plus, they're slightly sticky, which means that they trap skin flakes where they'll be most visible. So if dandruff is a problem, use sprays and gels sparingly—if at all.

Get the right shampoo. Dandruff shampoos purchased over the counter will reduce the rate at which skin cells grow and die, which, in turn, means less flaking. They'll also combat that pesky yeast. Look for shampoos containing selenium sulfide (Selsun Blue or Head & Shoulders) or zinc pyrithione (X-Seb or Zincon). Massage the shampoo into your scalp for at least a minute. Rinse. Then rub in some more, says Richard S. Berger, M.D., clinical professor of dermatology at the University of Medicine and Dentistry of New Jersey, Robert Wood Johnson Medical School in Piscataway, New Jersey.

Make the switch. If you've been successfully using a dandruff shampoo but your dandruff has suddenly made a new appearance, it could be time to switch shampoos. The reason is that yeasts on your scalp can build up resistance to certain shampoos. If you switch to another shampoo with a different ingredient, you can outsmart them, says Dr. Berger. For instance, if you are using a shampoo with selenium sulfide, switch to one with zinc pyrithione, coal tar (Tegrin or MG217) or salicylic acid (Neutrogena Healthy Scalp, P&S Shampoo, or MG217 Tar Free) instead.

Ease the inflammation. Doctors often recommend hydrocortisone ointments for treating mild psoriasis. More severe forms can be treated with ultraviolet light at some doctors' offices. Psoriasis causes skin to lose water, so lubricating your scalp with olive oil can help soothe the rash, says Dr. Stickler.

Dr. Kitzmiller recommends that you massage olive oil onto your scalp, wrap your hair in a towel for about ten minutes, remove the towel and shampoo. However, this severe treatment is usually only recommended if the scalp is very crusty.

Itchy Skin

• Your skin is dry and cracked

What It ? Means

Your body detects an itchy feeling in the middle of your right shoulder blade. Your left arm reaches over your right shoulder. Almost. Almost. Almost.

Damn. It doesn't reach.

Your right arm cranks behind the back. Just a little higher. Closer. Closer.

Ahhh. Got it.

Bliss.

Only now the itch has wandered toward the middle of your back, and you'd have to un-screw your arm to reach it.

Itchy skin is a torment. And the obvious solution—scratching—seems to make things even more itchy. It's not your imagination. Scratching one itch excites other nerves nearby, causing them to itch as well, says Dr. Mitchell C. Stickler of Lewes, Delaware.

What makes us itch in the first place? Usually, it's dry skin, particularly in the cold months. Cold air contains less water vapor than warm air. Heaters remove additional moisture from the air, making the skin even drier, says Dr. Stickler. In winter, the skin loses more moisture to this dry air, causing dry, itchy skin.

Other itch-makers include rashes, insect bites, stress and even internal diseases, such as cancer. (For additional information on itching, see Rashes on page 137.)

Symptom Solver

First of all, don't scratch. It's not good for your skin. "In fact, if you concentrate on scratching a small area of your skin religiously for five minutes a day, at the end of the month you would have a nice little thickened area of skin called localized neurodermatitis," says Dr. K. William Kitzmiller of the University of Cincinnati.

Since it's so hard not to scratch, however, it's best to eliminate the itch. Here's how.

Ice the itch. Putting a cold compress on an itchy spot such as a mosquito bite will slow nerve signals so that the area won't feel as itchy, says Dr. Kitzmiller.

Get some fatty acids. Since your body doesn't manufacture essential fatty acids, you have to get them from your diet in foods such as cold-water fish and flaxseed. Or you can take a fatty-acid supplement, available at many health food stores. These acids help lubricate your eyes, skin and throat, says Robert Abel, Jr., M.D., clinical professor of ophthalmology at Thomas Jefferson University in Philadelphia.

When taking fatty-acid supplements, start with the lowest dosage. Take it for a month and see if it helps. Then increase the dosage if you need to, Dr. Abel advises.

Stay cool and dry. When water evaporates from your skin, it leaves you parched. Hot water tends to be particularly drying. So it's a good idea to keep showers and baths short and not too hot—especially in winter when the air is dry, says Dr. Stickler.

Limit the suds. Soap dries the skin, so don't overdo it. Use it mainly to wash your face, armpits, genitals and feet, Dr. Stickler says. And use a mild soap such as Oil of Olay, Dove or Basis, or a soapless cleanser like Cetaphil lotion.

Be slippery when wet. Applying a moisturizer while your skin is still wet will help lock in moisture. Smooth it over your entire body, not just your face and hands. "Your legs need more cold-weather moisturization because they have fewer sebaceous glands to lubricate them naturally," says Amy E. Newburger, M.D., assistant clinical professor of dermatology at Columbia University School of Medicine in New York City.

You don't have to spend a lot of money on a moisturizer. They all do pretty much the same thing, Dr. Stickler says.

Moles

• Pink, dark brown or black skin growths

What It ? Means

Though moles can be unsightly, they usually pose no threat. But they aren't good for anything either. "We would do just fine without them," says Dr. Mitchell C. Stickler of Lewes, Delaware.

While most moles are good for nothing, the bad ones are bad to the bone. Moles called atypical can be precancerous. That means that they are more likely to turn into a melanoma, a deadly form of cancer. Melanomas have doubled in frequency over the past 20 years, possibly an ominous sign of the loss of the protective ozone layer. The most rapid increase of melanomas has occurred in older men—usually on their heads and necks.

You can recognize an atypical mole by its irregular border, variations in color and its irregular shape. Any mole that has an irregular shape or color or that is larger than a quarter-inch across should be considered potentially dangerous. Any mole that appears to be changing should be looked at by a doctor, recommends Dr. Stickler.

The average white person has 25 to 40 moles. Darker-skinned people have fewer. Most moles are formed during the first two decades of life, enlarging as the person grows. They are most common on the parts of your body that get the most sun, like on your neck and shoulders. The number of moles you have depends on heredity and how much time you spend in the sun, says Dr. Stickler.

Symptom Solver

If your moles are the healthy, run-of-the-mill kind, you don't need to do anything, says Dr. Stickler. If they make you uncomfortable, you can have a doctor remove them.

There are two surgical options for removing moles. You can have the protruding part shaved off. But that leaves the root and discoloration intact; there's a chance that the mole will rear an even uglier head in the future. Or you can have the entire mole removed. The problem here is that the surgery may leave a scar that looks worse than the mole.

Atypical moles are always a serious matter. Here's what to do.

Keep them in check. You should regularly inspect moles to see if they're growing or changing shape or color. In addition, it's a good idea to have your doctor look them over once a year, especially if anyone in your family has had a melanoma, says Dr. Stickler. Moles need to be looked at by a doctor immediately if they change in color, size or shape or if they bleed or itch.

Stay in the shade. Sunlight is thought to be the biggest cause of melanoma. You would think that people who work outside for a living would have the highest risk of melanoma. But that's not entirely true. It's the guy who works inside all week then goes to the beach for the weekend who has the most to worry about. People who spend a lot of time in the sun have a higher rate of other types of skin cancer, like basal cell and squamous cell cancers. It's people who are exposed to sunlight sporadically who have the highest rates of melanoma, the deadliest type of skin cancer, says Dr. Stickler.

When spending time outdoors, always wear a sunscreen with a sun protection factor (SPF) of 15 or more. And don't think that just because you're wearing a shirt that the sun's not getting to your skin. The SPF of a wet, cotton T-shirt is only about a 2 or 3. So wear sunscreen underneath, says Nicholas J. Lowe, M.D., professor of dermatology at the University of California, Los Angeles, School of Medicine. And avoid spending time in the sun between 10:00 A.M. and 2:00 P.M., when the intensity of the rays is greatest.

Rashes

• Any eruption or breakout on the skin

What It ? Means

The problem with rashes is that there are so many of them. We're talking about 10,000 or more. So they are kind of hard to self-diagnose.

But some rashes are more common than others. So here are descriptions of some of the more common rashes.

•Allergic rashes. If you eat something that your body doesn't like, hives—red, swollen bumps surrounded by a white halo—can suddenly cover all or part of your body. Hives caused by a food allergy usually disappear within 24 hours. It can be very difficult to pinpoint the cause.

Another type of allergic rash occurs when you brush against something your skin doesn't like, like poison ivy, poison sumac or poison oak. Although each of these plants can cause a bubbly, itchy, yucky rash, they really aren't poisonous. Most people are simply allergic to their resin. The allergy builds over time. So the first time you brush up against poison ivy, you might escape rash-free. Later, after repeated exposures, you may find yourself breaking out. Or not. It all depends whether you're susceptible to that type of allergy.

You don't have to come in direct contact with the plant to be affected. You can get it from a dog that has rubbed up against a plant or from clothing that has. The rash doesn't occur right away but can take anywhere from four hours to ten days before breaking out. The rash itself is not contagious, even though the liquid-filled blisters that it causes make it look that way.

•Sweat rashes. Prolonged sweating can clog your sweat ducts. Then the duct breaks open and sweat leaks beneath the skin, causing pores to swell into red bumps. The medical name for the condition is miliaria, though most people call it prickly heat or heat rash.

Another sweat-related rash is Grover's disease, which usually affects white men older than 40. It causes small red bumps on the chest, stomach, back and sometimes the arms and legs. Though the cause is unknown, the rash is associated with sun exposure, heat and sweating.

•Irritated rashes. Your hands are prime candidates for this. The use of harsh soaps coupled with the dry air of winter can make the skin on your hands really parched and sore. Throw in some bare-handed snow shoveling and you have some really dry skin to contend with.

•Bug-induced rashes. Various creatures can burrow into the skin or give a bite and cause a rash. Chiggers are a common cause of rashes. These tiny red insects are usually herbivores. But when they see you coming, they think, "Yum, protein." They aim for areas where the skin is thin, like on the ankles, wrists, thighs, groin and waist. When feeding, they inject some saliva. And that's what causes a mean rash in some people.

Symptom Q Solver

If your rash occurs with a fever, you should see a doctor. Otherwise there are a few remedies that help most rashes.

Soothe with cortisone cream. Available over the counter and by prescription, this powerful medication can help ease rashes fast. You can use it for up to three days, says Dr. Mitchell C. Stickler of Lewes, Delaware. If the rash doesn't get better by then, see a doctor.

Call for icing. Cold compresses will soothe hives and other rashes as well as suppress the itch, says Dr. K. William Kitzmiller of the University of Cincinnati. An ice pack works well. Or you can wrap ice cubes in a damp washcloth and apply the compress to the area for 15 minutes.

Have some soda. Baking soda can help relieve the itching caused by rashes by temporarily changing the pH of the skin from acid to alkaline, says Leonard Grayson, M.D., chief of the Department of Allergy and Dermatology at Quincy Medical Group in Quincy, Illinois. Make a paste by adding a little water to the baking soda, then smooth the concoction over the rash. Or simply add the baking soda to cool bath water and soak in it.

Sow your oats. Soaking in an oatmeal bath can help relieve itchy rashes, according to one study. Use a colloidal oatmeal, such as Aveeno. Sprinkle it in the tub as it is filling, then soak for 20 minutes. Repeat twice a day.

Try chamomile. Either rub some chamomile extract onto the skin or apply gauze that's been soaked in strong, cooled chamomile tea, recommends Varro E. Tyler, Ph.D., professor of pharmacognosy at Purdue University School of Pharmacy in West Lafayette, Indiana.

Take fast action. If you've just touched poison oak, poison ivy or another poisonous plant, washing with a strong soap soon after contact may help prevent an outbreak. If you can, wash with a 5 percent solution of hydrogen peroxide and water instead of soap.

Stop the sweat. To prevent sweat rashes, you need to avoid excessive heat and humidity. Wear loose cotton clothing, take cool baths and use air-conditioning. Applying

Cetaphil lotion, available over the counter, several times a day will help relieve irritation resulting from many rashes, says Dr. Stickler.

Pamper your hands. Whenever you garden, handle acidic foods or use irritants such as detergents and paint thinners, wear waterproof, cotton-lined gloves to avoid rashes, Dr. Stickler says. When washing your hands, use lukewarm water and a small amount of mild soap such as Dove or Basis. Rinse the soap off carefully and dry gently.

Avoid that bug. When walking in areas filled with low brush, keeping your skin covered will help prevent buggy "hitchhikers" from catching a ride. It's also a good idea to apply insect repellent containing dimethyl phythalate (Off! Skintastic), Dr. Stickler says.

Say good-bye to hives. Diphenhydramine (Benadryl) and other over-the-counter antihistamines will usually help control hives within a few days or sooner. When the problem persists, however, or if you're having trouble breathing, see a doctor right away, Dr. Stickler says. It's also a good idea to avoid aspirin and other nonsteroidal anti-inflammatory medications like ibuprofen and codeine, all of which can make hives worse.

The Noxious Threesome

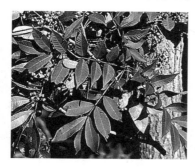

Poison sumac. **The leaves are divided into 7 to 13 leaflets. Each leaflet is pointed and smooth-edged. The stalks to the leaves are reddish. It is usually found in wet, swampy areas.**

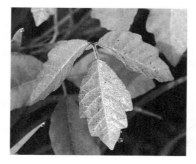

Poison oak. **The leaves are three-part, and the plant has flowers and fruit that hang in clusters. The berrylike fruit is yellow or white. Like poison ivy, it's found in many parts of the United States.**

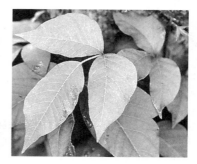

Poison ivy. **It can be a climbing vine or low, bushy shrub and is adorned with three-part, pointed leaves. The leaves are shiny and have toothed edges. It's found throughout the United States.**

Unwanted Hair Growth

• Hairs are sprouting wildly in embarrassing places: ears, nose and eyebrows

• You feel like Lon Chaney, Jr., during a full moon, as hair creeps over your back and shoulders

What It ? Means

For men, the laws of hair growth are probably the cruelest of all.

As we age, we tend to lose hair where we want it—on top of our heads—and gain it where we don't—in our nostrils, ears and eyebrows. Doctors aren't really sure why it happens. But the extra bristles usually make themselves noticeable at about age 50 and really get bushy during your sixties and seventies.

Plus, there's a double whammy: Men who tend to lose hair on top are the same guys who usually have lots of it elsewhere, like on their shoulders and backs. That's because testosterone, the hormone responsible for hair loss on the head, is also responsible for hair growth elsewhere on the body.

To some extent how hairy you are depends on your basic genetic stock. Men with excessive body hair can usually trace their ancestry to a place where people tend to be hairy, such as the Middle East, says Ken Hashimoto, M.D., professor and chairman of the Wayne State University School of Medicine in Detroit.

You may not want the extra hair, but it's hard to argue with your genes. For some men, hairiness is just a normal part of life, says Dr. Hashimoto.

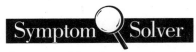

Symptom Solver

If you would rather that the hair today was gone tomorrow, then here are some suggestions.

Shave it. The easiest way to get rid of hair growing on the outside of your ears is to extend your shaving territory. Moisten your ear and gently work the razor around the lobe and outer leaf, or wherever the hair is growing. Don't worry about the hair growing back thicker. It's a myth. "It will grow back, but it absolutely will not grow back thicker," says John Romano, M.D., a dermatologist with New York Hospital-Cornell Medical Center in New York City.

Get some help. Your barber can trim up your ear and nose with an electric trimmer and some shears. Don't worry; he's not going to stick anything up your nose. He's just going to clip the visible hairs that are growing out of the nostrils and ears, says Okoye Morgan, a barber and trichologist—an expert in the scientific study of hair—at Sam's Barber Shop in St. Petersburg, Florida.

Be careful with scissors. Electric clippers are much safer than scissors when it comes to hair removal in noses and ears. "Most people who use scissors end up cutting themselves," says Dr. Romano.

If you do use scissors, make sure that they are small, blunt-tipped grooming scissors, suggests Morgan. It's a good idea to ask someone with a steady hand and a clear line of sight to do the job, suggests Tom Easton of The Body Shop.

Clip that brow. Women tweeze unwanted eyebrow hair. The problem is that it can make the eyes tear and the nose run. You don't need to suffer that way, Morgan says. Use a comb to pull out and isolate the hairs you want to get rid of. Then clip them off with scissors or buzz them off with an electric razor. That way, you'll leave the general shape of the eyebrow intact.

Warts

- Small, skin-color bump or cluster of bumps

- Shape and texture varies, depending on where you get them

What It Means

Remember Dryfus, that snot-nosed, whiny-voiced, knotty-haired kid who followed you everywhere? You tried your hardest to ditch him. One day you even tied him to a tree way back in the woods. But just as you were walking into your yard feeling like a free boy, there was Dryfus, tugging at your sleeve, asking you to play that cowboys and Indians game again.

That little wart.

Now you have something on your skin that sort of reminds you of Dryfus: a wart. Dryfus and the wart share a key characteristic: It's almost impossible to ditch them.

Caused by a virus, warts start out as small, skin-color masses that eventually turn into rough little bumps. Warts can grow on any part of your body. They vary in appearance depending on their location. On the bottom of the foot they are usually firm and rough. On the hands they are usually bumpy with tiny black dots in the middle—the capillaries that bring them blood. On the face they are usually flat and clustered.

Wherever they grow, warts are extremely unpredictable. Some people attract warts like crazy. Others could probably roll around in warts and never get one of their own. Doctors don't really know why. It's one of those unexplained mysteries of life. Some people attract Dryfuses, too.

The virus that causes warts is contagious. But you can't avoid it. It might linger on computer keyboards, toilet paper dispensers or doorknobs. You can get it simply from holding someone's hand. And it may take months after exposure for the wart to appear.

Most warts are harmless. If you cut them, they'll bleed. But the odds are that they won't turn into cancer. Plantar warts, however, which grow on the sole of the foot, can be painful from all the pressure. Only in very rare cases have untreated plantar warts become cancerous.

Symptom Solver

There are tons of wart treatments. But none work all the time. Whatever you decide to do has a 70 percent chance of working, including doing nothing.

Here are a few things you may want to try, says Dr. Mitchell C. Stickler of Lewes, Delaware.

Do a slow burn. You can buy anti-wart preparations at the drugstore. Look for one that contains at least 15 percent salicylic acid or 15 percent lactic acid (Wart-Off, Duofilm, Duoplant Gel). These are chemicals that will slowly burn away the wart.

Some preparations involve sticking a pad on the wart and leaving it there for several days while the medication works. Or you can use a brush and apply liquid medication directly to the wart every evening, using a file between applications to help wear it down. Either way, it's a slow process. It may take a few months for the wart to disappear.

Corral them. Like most viral ailments, warts are contagious. You should not share clothing or linens with someone who has them. If you have penile warts, be sure to wear a condom to prevent transmission during intercourse.

Get professional help. There are many things that your doctor can do to remove warts, ranging from freezing them with liquid nitrogen to burning them off with lasers. But medical treatments can be mucho expensive. And in some people the wart can grow right back.

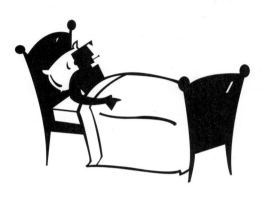

Part Eight

Real-Life Scenarios

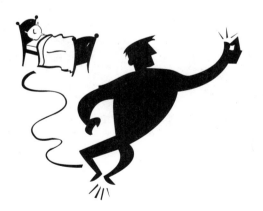

Quest for the Best
They're world-beaters: successful, celebrated and at the top of their games. But they're not invincible. Like many men, they've had to face serious health problems and are now stronger and wiser for the experience. Here are their stories.

You Can Do It!
These guys face the same pressures as you—juggling jobs, families and other important responsibilities. They also have had to face specific health concerns—some major, some relatively minor. As a result, they have learned to take control of their health, and you can, too.

Road Map to Health
Your health needs are different at age 50 than they are at age 20. So what you need is a decade-by-decade program that spells out precisely which tests need to be done and which health problems are likely to crop up. Here it is.

Quest for the Best
They're world-beaters: successful, celebrated and at the top of their games. But they're not invincible. Like many men, they've had to face serious health problems and are now stronger and wiser for the experience. Here are their stories.

Charles M. Harper, Former Chairman and Chief Executive Officer, RJR Nabisco

Making a Healthy Choice

When Charles M. Harper suffered a heart attack in September 1985, it appeared that he was faced with a choice: He could either go on eating the way that he always had and dig himself an early grave, or he could cut out the high-fat foods that he loved and resign himself to a long—and bland—life.

Some choice. But luckily for Harper, a third option came along—a Healthy Choice. And it revolutionized the frozen-foods industry.

Like many lifelong midwesterners, Harper—who was the head of ConAgra, an agribusiness giant based in Omaha, Nebraska, at the time of his heart attack—considered beef to be one of the essential food groups. "I loved to eat anything greasy, probably the greasier the better," he recalls longingly.

But he can't, not since his heart attack more than ten years ago. At the time, Harper's cholesterol level fluctuated around 260—60 points above what's considered normal and 20 points above what's considered high.

Harper, who was in his late fifties at the time, wasn't about to go on a low-fat, might-as-well-not-have-any-taste-buds

diet. He needed an alternative. And fortunately for him, he didn't have to look any further than his own kitchen to find one.

Cooking Up a Plan

When doctors told Harper to forfeit the fat or his life, he envisioned a small section of the grocery store that sold nuts and twigs. It wasn't an appetizing thought. But Josie, his wife, hit on a better idea. She simply substituted ground turkey for beef. That way, she could cook meals that didn't sacrifice the ingredient Harper loved most—meat.

Josie cooked one low-fat dish after another. There was turkey meat loaf. Turkey burgers. Turkey chili. And fortunately for the rest of us, Harper—as chairman of ConAgra—was in a position to put healthy foods on grocery store shelves.

"I was at home recuperating, and we had the head of ConAgra marketing come out to have lunch with me," Harper says. "My wife served chili made with turkey. He and I both remarked about how shocked we were that there can be something that is probably good for you

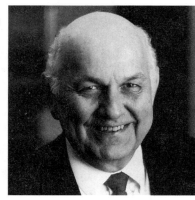

that tastes good. So the whole notion of something that tasted great that still was good for you and low-fat was born right there."

Three years later, ConAgra launched Healthy Choice frozen dinners, the first low-fat, low-salt frozen-dinner line. It was food that Harper could eat and, even more important, food that he would want to eat. Today, the Healthy

Choice brand brings in $1 billion annually in retail sales.

"It took lots of smart people, not including myself," Harper says. "I give all the credit to Josie, though."

After the frozen dinners came Healthy Choice cheese. Then Healthy Choice pasta sauce. And Healthy Choice soup and luncheon meats. When Harper travels—which is much of the workweek—he eats it all.

He eats grilled cheese sandwiches made with nonfat Healthy Choice cheese, burgers made from Swift 95 Supreme extra lean ground beef, Butterball turkey bacon and Butterball meat loaf. "I love sausage. And, of course, sausage is very high on the no-no list if you're thinking about fat. But if you have a turkey sausage, that's really not bad for you," says Harper.

Every once in a long while (he jokes that it's every hundred years, but it only seems that way), Harper treats himself to those greasy french fries. "I don't think that it's killed me yet," he quips.

Rising to the Top

Harper grew up in Lansing, Michigan, graduated from Purdue University in West Lafayette, Indiana, and moved on to the University of Chicago for his master's degree. After working as an engineer at General Motors, Harper became a group vice-president at Pillsbury before assuming the reins at ConAgra in 1974.

When he arrived, ConAgra was financially troubled from bad investments and commodity speculation. Harper reduced debt by trimming properties and got the company back in shape by 1977. In 1978 ConAgra bought United Agri Products, which manufactures agricultural chemicals.

It was the first of a series of acquisitions that included Banquet frozen foods, Singleton Seafood, Sea-Alaska, Country Pride, Armour Food Company and RJR Nabisco's frozen-foods lines, such as Chung King, Morton, Beatrice

Foods and many other trademarks. Such acquisitions helped ConAgra to acquire the top-selling popcorn (Orville Redenbacher's) and the number one tomato sauce (Hunt's).

His success with ConAgra made Harper an extremely valuable commodity in his own right, and in 1993, after his retirement as ConAgra's chief executive officer, he was acquired by RJR Nabisco, a manufacturer of consumer goods, including Snackwell's, the popular low-fat product. Harper is the former chairman and chief executive officer.

A Man of Taste

For Harper, life after a heart attack doesn't mean a life without pleasure.

He admits that he should exercise a bit more. And though he wouldn't tell us how much he actually weighs, he conceded that his doctor would like him to lose a few pounds.

"I have focused on low fat. I don't exercise as much as I should. But I've been pretty religious about low fat," Harper says. "I don't pass on meat. I'll have veal and turkey—turkey meat loaf, turkey sausage, turkey burgers. There's a hamburger that ConAgra makes that is extraordinarily low in fat but made with beef. And it doesn't taste like a piece of cardboard.

"I don't believe that people are going to eat anything that's good for them unless it tastes great. They are not going to make the sacrifice of poor eating quality just for low fat."

The low-fat diet has helped him keep his cholesterol down without the use of medication. His cholesterol level is now in the 170 to 180 range.

Harper says that finding a way to eat the foods he loves has helped him stay happy as well as healthy. Substituting lower-fat versions of his favorite foods keeps him from feeling like he's living a life of quiet deprivation.

"I haven't changed my diet except in the composition of it," Harper says. "I eat the same kinds of things, so how can I get a craving? I'm getting satisfied for the same things that I had before."

Michael Olajidé, Jr., Former World Middleweight Contender

Finding Life outside the Ring

It's the beginning of the sixth round, and by all accounts, the most important fight of Michael Olajidé, Jr.'s, life is not going as planned. His strategy for wresting the World Boxing Organization super middleweight championship belt from Thomas Hearns is simple: Avoid going toe-to-toe with the Hitman. Don't trade punches. Just stick and move and wear him out. And wait for an opportunity.

"In retrospect, it may not have been the smartest way to go," Olajidé now says of his 1990 title bout. "I gave him so many points. By that stage of the fight, I had backed myself into a corner. I really needed to take it to him."

The bell rings. The fighters trade punches. At some point, Hearns connects with a jab to Olajidé's right eye, which still has not completely recovered from a detached retina. Not a devastating blow by any means. But it's enough.

As the rounds wear on, the intensity of both fighters steadily increases. In the ninth round, Hearns hits Olajidé with a right that drops him. Olajidé staggers to his feet and signals to the referee that he's ready to continue. The problem is that he isn't sure where the punch came from; the world as seen through his right eye is now a blur. Miraculously, Olajidé responds with a shot that rocks Hearns at the bell.

Tenth round. Olajidé connects again. Hearns knows that he's in trouble. He starts moving. And Olajidé spends the rest of the night trying to find

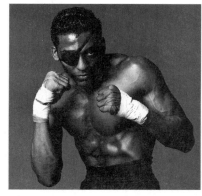

him—literally. "That's when I really recognized there was a serious problem with my eye," he says. "My depth perception really hurt me. I couldn't find him in terms of range. I was throwing punches that weren't even near him." Hearns wins a unanimous decision easily. *Sports Illustrated* calls it a lopsided victory.

"Had I won that fight, it would have been Sugar Ray Leonard and I at the Garden," Olajidé says wistfully.

Eye of the Tiger

Instead, Olajidé found himself at a New Jersey eye doctor's office desperate for a treatment that would allow him to fight again. "Boxers have this aura about them, like they think they are invincible or something—even if it is false. You just think, 'It will never happen to me. The other guy got knocked out, but it won't happen to me,' " he says.

For the first few golden years of Olajidé's career, it *didn't* happen to him. His smooth style earned him the nickname The Silk. At the age of 23, the soft-spoken, English-born fighter was 23–0, ranked in the top ten, a favorite of the New York media and—as if all that wasn't enough—moonlighted as a model.

Not bad for a kid who wandered into his father's Vancouver boxing gym for the first time at age 15 skinny as a stick. A professional fighter himself, the elder Olajidé immediately stood his son in front of a full-length mirror and taught him how to jab. "I was sore from the repetitiveness of the punch, pumping it out and back, out and back," Olajidé later recalled in a book written with former *New York Times* journalist Phil Berger.

Daddy's training served him well. By 1987, Olajidé was the number one contender for Marvin Hagler's International Boxing Federation middleweight title—a shot he probably would have received if Hagler hadn't been offered much bigger money to fight the ever-popular Sugar Ray Leonard.

But even as Olajidé's star rose—legendary fight trainer Angelo Dundee signed on the year before the Hearns fight—his right eye took a beating. And when Hearns re-injured it, his options were simple. He could quit boxing or see if he could get it fixed.

Olajidé wasn't ready to quit. So the doctor went to work, repairing the damage to his eye with something called a scleral buckle. "Normally, when you have a detached retina, they put on this buckle that goes around the eye completely. But what this doctor did was put on one that only went around half the eye. And so two ends were protruding from the ball, pushing against it like a knife or a pin under material," he says.

An End—And a Beginning

Four months later, Olajidé traveled to Alabama, where—without an athletic commission to sanction the bout—he climbed back into the ring against a 41-year-old journeyman named Ralph Moncrief. "It was one of these comeback fights—one where you want to test it out to see if it works," he says.

It didn't. Olajidé took a beating, and his trainer threw in the towel in the eighth round. "When I got hit, the buckle punctured the retina walls, and the fluid leaked out. At that point I almost lost the eye," says Olajidé. "The doctor said that I would never see normally out of it again. I was fully responsible and should have been aware of these things. But sometimes you just don't have a sense of . . . I don't know . . . mortality. You walk around like nothing can happen to you, and it did."

In 1991, at age 27, Olajidé was forced to retire from the only career he had ever known. His final record was 27–4. While some might have grown bitter or angry or both, Olajidé got busy. While trying to figure out what he was going to do with the rest of his life, he began

working with New York City physical therapist, Daniel Hamner, M.D., who was looking for a way to give his patients a good upper body workout while their shinsplints and knee problems healed. Olajidé had the answer: a boxing workout—without the opponent.

A short time later, Olajidé was approached about teaching one-on-one boxing at the Crosby Street Gym. Olajidé was interested but had a different plan in mind. "I knew that the one-on-one training was very strenuous. People miss the pads and want to hit you. They want to spar with you. So I said, 'Geez, I've been hit enough in my life. All I need is to get hit, have some kind of flashback, deck somebody, and I'll be sued forever,' " he recalls, laughing.

Instead, Olajidé suggested that he teach boxing fundamentals such as the jab, uppercut, hook and footwork as if it were an aerobics class. *Aerobox* was born. It was an instant hit at the Crosby Street Gym, and Olajidé soon took the routine to two other New York fitness clubs.

Along the way, Olajidé—now sporting an eye patch—teamed with fitness queen Kathy Smith to choreograph and star in a workout video called *Aerobox Workout*. He also teamed with Berger to write a how-to workout book called *Aerobox: A High-Performance Fitness Program (The Ultimate Noncontact Boxing Workout)*.

"*Aerobox* is a workout that builds aerobic capacity while giving a sense of the movement of boxing. Guys love it because it's got the macho act of firing punches and the same bob and weave that pros do to elude punches. . . . Women love the workout for the intricacy of the movement," he says.

"Everything I do right now is so focused on boxing. I feel that it's been a great discipline. And because it's still so undeveloped, I've been able to come up with a few concepts that have helped me. I mean, this is what I did my whole life. I couldn't come out and be a computer specialist or nuclear scientist. But let me do what I know I do best," says Olajidé.

"What can I say? God loves a trier."

Mark Conover, Olympic Marathoner

Gaining a New Perspective on Life

Sitting at a bar next to two women, Mark Conover reached up to his head, grabbed a wad of hair and pulled it away from his scalp.

"Boy," he remarked, looking at the clump of hair in his fist. "I have to quit my job. It's way too much stress."

Even when the grueling chemotherapy treatments for cancer caused him to lose his hair, the former U.S. Olympic marathoner never lost his sense of humor. Or his positive outlook on life.

Take that barroom incident, for example. His little stunt sparked a conversation with the two women, one of whom told Conover how she had dealt with the discovery of an ovarian cyst. "People are equally vulnerable and have their stories to tell," says Conover, who lives in San Luis Obispo, California. "If you can be open about it, you can grow."

Feeling Run-Down

Conover, now in his mid-thirties, came out of nowhere to win the U.S. Olympic marathon trials in 1988. It was while training for the trials four years later that Conover first realized that something was wrong.

"About two months before that race, I just started getting a lot of colds and the flu. I just attributed it to being run-down from the training," Conover recalls.

Conover ran that marathon but finished tenth. He continued to race, but the colds persisted. "By about June 1992, my energy was not quite right. My ability to do any hard training was starting to go down the drain. I would do a hard workout and catch a cold that

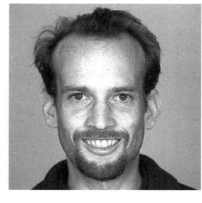

would last two to three days. I would think that I was better and go run again. Then I would get sick. The same thing just kept happening."

As the year wore on, Conover grew increasingly fatigued. A running friend who also was a doctor noticed that he wheezed as he ran. He suggested that Conover get checked for asthma and allergies. Doctors gave Conover various medications, but nothing seemed to work. As a precaution, they took x-rays of his lungs; however, nothing unusual turned up.

All the while Conover kept touching the lymph nodes in his neck. They seemed to be growing. "I thought, well, I'm just a skinny guy, and things stick out of my body anyway. I didn't really think anything of it," Conover says. And he didn't bring it to his doctor's attention.

By late 1993, Conover was so chronically tired that he gave up the idea of any intense running. Then in October, the weekend after he was inducted into his alma mater Humboldt State University's Sports Hall of Fame in Arcata, California, Conover got night sweats. His gastrointestinal tract seemed to have gone haywire. And an eerie sound came out of his throat when he breathed—a crackling noise.

"That weekend my health just really got worse. I went to my doctor, and I said, 'There's something really wrong here.' He felt the lymph nodes in my neck and noticed that one was really large. He sent me off to a pulmonary specialist," Conover says.

Conover again had his lungs x-rayed. As he drove to see the pulmonary specialist, he read the report by the x-ray technician. The report said not to rule out the possibility of lymphoma. "Lymphoma?" Conover wondered to himself.

He got to the doctor's office a little early. So he went to a library and looked up information on lymphoma and Hodgkin's disease. "By the time I got to the doctor, I pretty much knew that he would tell me that I had Hodgkin's disease. But it didn't really prepare me. When he said it, I just went numb and cried," says Conover. "There also was a sense of relief. When you are a runner and the body is not responding, you wonder if it's all in your head. This validated that years of problems were definitely not all in my head."

Driving home from the doctor's office that day, Conover stopped at a traffic light. The former U.S. Olympic marathoner looked over at the car next to him and noticed that the couple inside was arguing. He wanted to roll down his window and tell them that whatever they were arguing about probably wasn't that important.

But he didn't.

Running for His Life

Once the numbness and the shock subsided, Conover looked at cancer as a challenge. He began a six-month, biweekly chemotherapy treatment. He opted for a high dose of chemotherapy and no radiation because doctors told him that radiation would wipe out his chances of running competitively.

After each chemotherapy session, he experienced nausea and his skin would tingle and burn. And he was dead tired. The nausea and skin discomfort lasted a day. The fatigue lasted three to four days. So he usually had one good week before he "had to go get pelted again."

Despite his fatigue, Conover ran throughout the treatment. "Running has been more of a therapy for me. It helped to get me through it. Even on my worst days, I had to go out and jog for 20 minutes. It was just so I knew that I was still living life and feeling the wind against my face."

At some point during the treatment, Conover's tumors shriveled up inside his lungs. And Conover has little worry that the cancer will return.

The fact that Conover lived to tell about his harrowing experience is not unusual. Hodgkin's disease is one cancer that is very curable. But Conover then did something that stunned much of the world. One year after fin-

ishing his chemotherapy, he qualified for the 1996 Olympic trials in the marathon.

"I don't even really think of myself as ever having been that severely sick just because I've been able to get back into running," Conover says. "If you can go out, no matter what kind of exercise you've done, and feel strong and healthy and vital, that'll be your mind-set. You won't be dwelling on your health problem. You'll be dwelling on what kind of workout you want to do tomorrow. If you can keep a good exercise routine, that mind-set takes over so that you don't really dwell on the fact that you were sick. At least that's what it did for me."

Conover still hasn't been able to regain the speed he had before his bout with cancer. At the trials he didn't come close to running a time that would have secured a spot on the U.S. Olympic team.

"It has been hard for me to get a lot of the speed back that I had in 1988 or 1992. I feel pretty good running, but I don't recover as well as I did back then. That could be a combination of factors, including the wear and tear of the chemotherapy."

Still, Conover looks at his cancer as a positive event in his life and as a learning experience.

"I think that anybody who goes through cancer will change his perspective on what really matters. He'll be able to look past the real trivial things that people worry about. You realize that you are not here for that long, so why live your life in unproductive patterns?

"I'm not saying that I have everything figured out in life," says Conover, who left his local government job to devote himself to coaching, freelance writing on various running publications and editing a local running magazine. "But you just look at the way that some people are living their lives, and you kind of know what level they are at. Cancer makes you feel perhaps a little wiser than most.

"I've said before that maybe everybody could use a small dose of cancer to help put things in perspective."

Bob Beamon, Olympic Gold Medalist

Soaring Over Hypertension

On a stormy day in October 1968, Bob Beamon sent an earth-shaking thunderclap through the world of track and field. In a sport where records are broken by tenths or hundredths of an inch, Beamon leapt nearly 2 feet beyond the existing world record to capture the gold medal for the United States in the Mexico City Olympics.

It was one of those feats that changes our understanding of what's possible and what's impossible. Before that day, no man had ever jumped 28 feet. Beamon, 22 at the time, obliterated that barrier, setting an incredible new standard of 29 feet 2½ inches that nobody would approach for the next 23 years.

Beamon was never able to jump that far again. But it was no fluke. His sports prowess dates back to his high school days. In fact, some of the records that he set at the time still stand today. In recognition of his achievements, Beamon—the National Collegiate Athletic Association long jump and triple jump champion in 1967—was inducted into the U.S. Olympic Committee Hall of Fame in 1992.

Ignoring the Signs

Young men tend to feel that they are invincible. And Beamon, a superbly conditioned, world-class athlete, certainly was no exception. So when his blood pressure started creeping up in his early thirties, Beamon largely ignored his doctor's advice to start paying attention to it. After all, the doctor didn't seem that worried about it. So neither was Beamon.

"I was in my thirties, and you kind of think, 'No big deal.' You are pretty much feeling your Cheerios. You think that you are too young to worry about health problems," Beamon says.

But as he neared his fortieth birthday, Beamon began to travel extensively to make celebrity appearances. And each time he flew, he suffered ear pain. Even well after landing, his ears would stay plugged. So just before one trip, he went to see his doctor to find out whether he could do anything about it.

As with any doctor's visit, the nurse took Beamon's blood pressure. But this reading was unlike any he had before—150 over 110. A reading of about 120 over 80 is considered normal.

This time, the doctor was very concerned. And so was Beamon.

A Familiar Story

Beamon grew up in the South Jamaica projects in Queens, New York. He was poor. Until age 14, he was illiterate. And he was the war counselor for his neighborhood gang.

But what really sticks out vividly in his mind about those teenage years is what was happening to the adult men in his neighborhood. Many had high blood pressure, also known as hypertension. In a way, they were a portrait of the larger world, where 38 percent of black men and one-third of white men have the disease. But the men in Beamon's neighborhood rarely sought out medical care. And one after another, they suffered debilitating strokes.

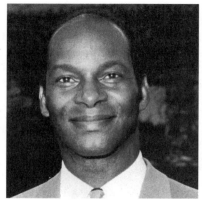

The 150-over-110 reading brought back those painful childhood memories. And Beamon realized that if he didn't change, he would be heading down the same road as the men from his old neighborhood.

"For the first time I became very concerned about my blood pressure, and my doctor was concerned about it. There was the possibility of becoming a stroke victim. I never paid too much attention to hypertension until that day. But then that day was it. As a matter of fact, I canceled my trip," says Beamon.

The doctor immediately gave him a shot to help lower his blood pressure and placed him on a medication regimen. Also, he gave up anything that could possibly interfere with his blood pressure or health in any way—cold turkey. He stopped drinking alcohol. He stopped salting his food. He stopped eating red meat.

"I used to drink beer and sometimes, depending on the occasion, a harder liquor. I gave it up. I just gave up everything. I stopped that day. I don't eat beef. I don't eat pork. I basically eat poultry and fish," Beamon says.

Those lifestyle changes paid off. Beamon now has his blood pressure under control, with the help of medication. Beamon isn't sure what caused his blood pressure to skyrocket. It could be part heredity, part lifestyle. But he hasn't really pondered it that much. He's not worried about the past. What's important to him is that he can live his life without the worry of stroke looming over his head.

Spreading the News

Beamon worries about other African-American men who ignore the blood pressure warning signs. For a while, Beamon served as a spokesman for a large pharmaceutical company to warn men about the connection between high blood pressure and strokes and heart attacks.

"In many cases men tend to not want to believe that high blood pressure is a silent killer," Beamon says. "African-Americans have a very high rate of hypertension. It's very interesting that black men shy away from medication. They worry about possible side effects. They worry that it may affect their energy levels and their attitudes. But they need to know that medicines have advanced quite a bit."

Beamon also wants to caution men about excessive drinking, including beer drinking. Though studies show that moderate alcohol consumption—about three beers a week—can actually help control high blood pressure, the key word is moderate. Excessive alcohol consumption has been linked to other health problems such as liver damage. And Beamon's message is simple: "In the long run it doesn't pay."

Search for Tomorrow

Beamon no longer frets about whether he'll end up incapacitated like one of the men from his old neighborhood. High blood pressure is just one of the many things that he has conquered.

It's his second major turnaround.

After conquering illiteracy as a teenager, Beamon went on to get a bachelor's degree in sociology and anthropology from Adelphi University in Garden City, New York.

Beamon's days of intense workouts and Olympic-caliber conditioning are behind him, but he still strives to stay fit. His exercise routine is more like cross-training—a combination of jogging, tennis and basketball—to manage stress and to keep healthy and happy. "It's great to go against the odds," Beamon says.

Today, Beamon works at creating programs to inspire youth and travels all over the world making appearances and speeches, carrying with him the motivating message, "Dare to Dream." He lives in Miami with his wife, Milana, and daughter, Deanna.

"I'm not going to worry. I know what I must do to remain healthy . . . it takes desire and discipline. I'd just like to be around to compete in the Senior Olympics one day," says Beamon.

You Can Do It! These guys face the same pressures as you—juggling jobs, families and other important responsibilities. They also have had to face specific health concerns—some major, some relatively minor. As a result, they have learned to take control of their health, and you can, too.

Fear Goes Up in Smoke

Greg Hrabar, Toms River, New Jersey

Date of birth: Feb. 22, 1948

Profession: Captain of the Jersey City Fire Department

It's easier for me to walk into a burning building than it is to walk up the steps to my dentist's office.

I've been trained to fight fires. I've been doing it for almost 24 years. Yeah, when the sirens are going and the flames are going and people are screaming, my heart thump, thump, thumps. But I've been there many times. I just go. I do what I have to do. It happens so quickly. One minute I'm sitting there or lying in bed, and three minutes later I'm hanging from a fire escape. There's no time to think.

But I've been scared of the dentist since I was about eight years old. I would wake up sweaty and shaky even the day before I had to go to the dentist. Back then, when I went to the dentist there would be a dozen people in the waiting room and a line stretched down the stairs. Mom would take me after school. And I could hear people in there screaming. If Mom wasn't sitting there saying, "Get in there," I would have been hoofing it out the door.

My mom made sure that I got to the dentist on a regular basis for most of my childhood. When I got to high school, I had to go by myself. But she was on top of me making sure that I got there.

Once I got to college she said, "You're a big boy now. Go on your own." I said, "Yeah, right." I stopped going to the dentist for almost five years.

It cost me a tooth.

On New Year's Eve during my senior year in college, I had such incredible pain in a tooth. I had been trying to nurse the tooth for a while. I had known something was wrong for about two months.

But I kept putting it out of my mind. I think that a filling had fallen out and I ignored it. That's not good. By New Year's Eve I was in so much pain that I was no longer able to deny it. This was something that I had to deal with. It wasn't getting any better.

Still, it was my girlfriend who forced me to go to the dentist. I went at noon on New Year's Eve. I had to have the tooth yanked. They said that it had to go. I was a little woozy. But I ended up going to a New Year's party that night.

Feeling Anxious

After losing that tooth, I figured that I better go back to the dentist on a regular basis before I lost all my teeth. One of the major reasons that I didn't like dentist's visits was that novocaine didn't work on me. My nerve endings were so hyper. By the time the novocaine would kick in, I would be home. I had already suffered through an extremely painful cavity filling.

But now my dentist and I have fixed that problem. Now I go and the dentist gives me gas to help calm me down about getting the needle. Then he gives me the needle. And

I sit in the waiting room for a half-hour until the novocaine kicks in.

But my dentist's visits still aren't easy. My fear of the dentist has to do with more than just pain. It's psychological. For instance, there was a scene from the Dustin Hoffman movie *Marathon Man* where there's an insane German dentist who is going to experiment on Hoffman. I couldn't watch it. I had to leave the movie theater. I did come back after the scene was over. But I had to get out of there.

Days before an appointment, I usually start feeling anxious. Because of that, I have to schedule my appointments for the first thing in the morning. That way I won't be thinking about it the whole day. If I scheduled an appointment in the afternoon, I would have all day to worry about it. And at some point during the day I would probably cancel my appointment.

Also, I try to make my appointments on a morning after I've worked a 24-hour shift at the fire department. That way I will be really tired—too tired to worry.

And my dentist gave me a prescription for anti-anxiety medication. I found that if I got up and took the medicine first thing in the morning before the appointment, I'd walk in there, he'd shoot me up and I would be able to do it.

Since I lost that tooth in college, I have gone to the dentist, more or less, on a regular basis. Every once in a while it stretches out to a year to a year and a half between appointments.

But I have a system. I usually let myself ignore my dentist's first six-month reminder to make an appointment. Then when I get the second six-month notice, I force myself to make an appointment.

Gumming Up the Works

Even though I've been going to the dentist fairly regularly since college, it was more recently that I began taking care of my teeth correctly.

Not too long ago, a bunch of guys at the firehouse were diagnosed with gum disease. They were all going through it at the same time and had to have corrective surgery. The guys at work know that I'm afraid of the dentist.

And with me being afraid of the dentist, when I heard their stories, I was scared. I didn't want to have to go through what they were going through. So when I went in to see the dentist, I asked about it. My dentist said that I had the very beginnings of gum disease. I caught it early. I've flossed religiously and used Listerine ever since. I don't want surgery, so I've been taking care of them.

When I was a kid, my philosophy was that my teeth were going to get punched out in a bar fight or while playing football or something. I wasn't really attached to them. So I didn't worry too much about taking care of them. I just thought, if my teeth fall out or a dentist has to yank them, fine. Then I found out that gum disease goes into the bone even after you lose your teeth. I was like, "Woo ah. Okay." That got me to take care of them.

Conquering the Fear

My fear of the dentist is something that I feel I have more or less conquered. I hate going. But I know that it's my mouth, and if I want to keep my teeth, I have to do it.

Since I'm no longer a kid, I know that having a cavity is not the worst thing that can happen to me. There are many other things that I can think of that are worse. So if the dentist tells me that a tooth has to go, I can deal with it.

For other guys who don't go to the dentist, I can commiserate. I can tell them that I know how they feel. But you need to go. You need to get over the fear. If you don't, you'll end up losing your teeth.

Coming to Grips with Cancer

Joe Dvorak, South Barrington, Illinois

Date of birth: Oct. 3, 1945

Profession: Real estate broker

Two years ago, I was reading an article about prostate cancer in *Prevention* magazine. The article said that people who have prostate cancer in their families are at a higher risk for the disease. My father is in his eighties and has prostate problems. I didn't have any symptoms. No urination problems. No burning. But when I went to my doctor to get my blood cholesterol checked, I asked him to do a prostate-specific antigen (PSA) test, a blood test that can detect prostate cancer.

I took the test. I went back to his office a couple days later and asked about my cholesterol test. My doctor said, "Well, your cholesterol is fine. But I'm very concerned about your PSA. It's elevated. It's 7.9." I said, "What does that mean?" I didn't really know what my prostate was or where it was. He said that the test indicated that I could have one of three things: an irritation, an infection or cancer. He told me to make an appointment right away at the hospital to have an ultrasound.

I had the ultrasound. The doctors said that my prostate was slightly enlarged, and they recommended a biopsy. They took six cores. A couple of days later, I got the results. Three of the six had cancer. I got three doctors' opinions. They all told me the same thing. They said that it's unusual for someone so young to have it. They told me that it was curable and that they felt we found it quite early. They all recommended that I have surgery.

I was concerned, but I was not overly alarmed. I started reading about it. I learned about the potential complications—the loss of bladder control and sexual functions. Still I de-

cided to go ahead with the surgery. I selected a doctor at Northwestern University Hospital in Chicago who was one of the well-known doctors that performed nerve-saving surgery. At no time was I really concerned that the cancer would be a problem after the surgery. I figured that once I had the operation, I wouldn't have to worry about cancer anymore.

I went in for surgery August 24, 1994. After I came out, I asked my doctor, "How did it go?" He said, "The surgery went well. We think we got it all." And I said, "What do you mean you *think* you got it all?" He explained that I had a high-grade tumor, which is the kind that can spread quickly. He said that it had begun breaking through the side of my prostate wall but probably hadn't spread. He said there was a 70 percent chance that they got it all.

Switching to a Low-Fat Diet

My surgeon recommended radiation therapy as an extra precaution. I got three more doctors' opinions. One of the other doctors I consulted was the oncologist at Northwestern. He advised against radiation. He said that it was not proven that in the stage that I was at that the radiation would give me any more protection. He recommended that I get a PSA test every three to four months. And that's what I decided to do. I go every four months and have my PSA checked at Northwestern. As long as it is not elevated, they are comfortable.

I recovered very quickly from the surgery. I was out of the hospital within four days and back to work in a week. I lost ten pounds. I was weak. It took me a while to regain control of my bladder. And the sexual function is taking longer. They told me it takes 16 to 24 months. It's coming back.

When I made the decision to not have radiation, I went to a nutritionist who specializes in cancer patients. His plan was radical. He wanted to change my diet 180 degrees.

No red meat. No poultry. No dairy products. No sugar. The only things that I could eat were vegetables, fruits, grains and seafood. I tried to cut back. He also gave me a regimen of high doses of vitamins and nutrients. It was extremely expensive, and I really wasn't overly comfortable with it.

So I went to another nutritionist. I'm basically on a low-fat diet now. I don't eat red meat. But I do eat chicken and turkey sparingly. I eat a lot of fruits, vegetables and grains, and I'm taking high doses of vitamins and some nutrients.

For a while I attended meetings held by a support group called Us, Too, for people with prostate cancer. When you first find out that you have it, you know nothing about the disease. I highly recommend the support group. You meet other people with the disease who have lots of information about treatments. And the meetings include doctors who speak and answer questions about the disease.

Paying Attention to Health

The experience has really changed my life completely. I have a different attitude about what's important. And I will say that I probably will never take my health for granted again. When you don't have a health concern, you go to work every day and live your life somewhat in a routine. Until that operation in 1994, I never spent a day in the hospital except the day that I was born. I never had anything serious at all. My grandparents all lived to be 90. So in my mind, I thought that I would live to be 80 to 90 years old. When this happened, I just couldn't believe it. When you're healthy, you hear the word *cancer*, but it goes in one ear and out the other. When I hear *cancer* now, it is a word piercing to me.

I consider myself an extremely fortunate person. I have told every customer, friend and family member that I highly recommend the PSA test. I feel an obligation to let people know

what I have gone through. If I find one person that I've told who goes in and finds the cancer, I feel that I've really done something.

Living Proof

I am a living example of why PSA tests are important. I had a full physical with a rectal exam and ultrasound two years before my PSA test. Neither indicated that I had cancer. I am kind of sorry and angry that when I had that complete physical they did not give me a PSA. If they had, it's possible that I would have caught the tumor in an earlier stage and it would have been contained. I wouldn't have to worry about cancer showing up again.

Every four months I have to go back and get tested. When I see my surgeon, he'll say, "Joe, how are you doing?" I'll say, "Doctor, I'm doing great. I'm great for about three months, three weeks and about four days— until I have to see you." We do the exam. He takes my blood. And the next day I have to call for the results. That is very nerve-racking waiting on the phone for a nurse to tell me whether I have cancer again. I look at my life in four-month increments.

I'm much more vigilant about my health care now. Since I've had my surgery, I've elected to have further tests. I had a full colonoscopy. I had an electrocardiogram. My wife, Carol, thinks that I'm a hypochondriac. But if there is something there, I want to know. I want to know early so that I can work on it. Before my surgery, I didn't go to the doctor as often as I should. My checkups were once every three to four years. And up until four years ago, I never had a rectal exam. That's very common with men.

I now realize that I have a lot to be thankful for. I have two wonderful children, a good marriage and a good career. I'm financially stable. Hopefully, the cancer will not come back.

Back from the Brink

Charlie Walker, New Castle, Delaware

Date of birth: July 29, 1958

Profession: Literacy program coordinator

I guess it was early in the summer of 1995 when I started having chest discomfort. At first I attributed it to smoking too much or just overdoing it. And as anyone my age might say, I thought that I was too young to have any real health problems.

But it was a long summer. And I was under a lot of pressure. I had just finished working a part-time summer school job, I was working in a youth literacy program part-time and even though I wasn't happy, I was still working at the newspaper.

Everyone knows that journalism is a stressful profession. I was the night city editor at *The News Journal* in Wilmington, Delaware, directing all the live and breaking news coverage. That meant that I was the last editor at the gate for everything that was in the paper the next day. Anyone in the newsroom will tell you that it is the hardest and the best place to be. It's an incredible feeling—the deadlines and the adrenaline. You get off on it. But the amount of human tragedy—even though you are a professional—it takes an emotional toll. You're tough and you're steely when you're in there working, but the multiple homicides and the child abuse and the horrific car accidents take their toll. It was the only job I'd had since I was 18, and I was burning out on it.

It's not good for your lifestyle either. I wasn't a raging alcoholic, but up until a year ago I would have a few drinks after work. That's just what you did. I had reached a point where I couldn't do that anymore. When you're young, you feel that you're invulnerable—impervious to damage.

On the other hand, I'm not unintelligent. I was aware of the risk factors. I have a history of heart problems in the family: My maternal grandmother died of a heart attack, and my maternal grandfather suffered several heart attacks. He had heart bypass surgery. There's diabetes in the family. Scary stuff.

A Wake-Up Call

So I went back to school a couple of years ago with the intention of getting out of journalism. And because of that, for the last couple years I was burning the candle at both ends. I reached the point where I was working in summer school from 8:00 A.M. to 1:00 P.M., coming home, having lunch, going to work at 2:30 P.M. and working until midnight or later. And my intakes went up: I started drinking more coffee and smoking more cigarettes, and, needless to say, I didn't exercise a lick. I didn't have time. And my diet . . . I never ate breakfast—just drank coffee and smoked. For lunch I'd eat anything I wanted—fast food, fried chicken, you name it. And I never thought about having vegetables or anything like that.

Then one day that summer, I had smoked even more cigarettes than usual and was standing outside of work with a friend when I said to him, "It feels like somebody just hit me in the chest with a baseball bat." But I still had to go back to work at the paper. There was no option—they discourage you from calling in or going home sick.

By the time I got back inside the paper, I felt disoriented—almost nauseated. I didn't black out, but I didn't know what the hell was going on. So I called my wife, Donna, and she said, "You better call a doctor." So it's 8:30 at night, and I called and described the symptoms to him. He said, "Hang up the phone (right now) and call an ambulance."

So I did exactly what they tell you not to do. I hung up the phone and called my wife and asked her to come get me. At this point I was tottering. I went downstairs and told some people that I was leaving. Someone said,

"What's wrong?" I didn't care. At this point I had to leave. As much as I honor my responsibilities, I knew that I had to go.

I only live a few minutes away from the newspaper, and she was there quickly. So I got in the car, and when we pulled up to the emergency room, I was really disoriented. I never lost consciousness, but it was like I was on drugs or something. I wasn't panicking, but I knew that something was really wrong. My chest was just heaving. I couldn't catch my breath. The doctors immediately grabbed me and got me in there, wired me up and got the electrocardiogram monitor on me and got an IV going. My heart rate was extremely high. They were worried that I was going to go into a worse form of arrest at that point. They gave me nitroglycerin every ten minutes or so under my tongue, trying to stabilize me. Everything was extremely out of whack.

Now, when you aren't getting any blood or oxygen to your heart, the cells die. They wheeled me into the cardiac intensive care unit and kept me up there and on medication for two or three days and then brought me back down. Then they ran a series of tests. The tests showed that there hadn't been a blockage—and I didn't lose any tissue. No portion of my heart muscle died—it just was an electrical malfunction of some kind. I had all the symptoms of someone experiencing a heart attack but didn't actually have one.

A New Life

It was an awakening. I said, "Okay, I'm lucky. I'm 37. Maybe lightening struck about three feet from me, and maybe next time it's not going to miss." I had my last cigarette that night. And for someone who smoked for 22 years, there's barely an hour that passes that I don't think about it. But I don't smoke anymore. And more than ever I wanted to leave the paper.

I had been volunteering with this literacy program, and the professor in charge had been promised some grant money to create another paid position. He kept telling me that as soon as he got the money, he was going to hire me. But I was like, that'd be nice, but I'm not going to pin all my hopes on some money that may never come through.

When he got the grant in early October, I jumped. I was gone from the paper in two weeks. And it's been a major difference for me.

I figure that I was drinking two pots of coffee, 12 to 15 cups, a day. Now I have probably two real cups of coffee a day—mixed in with about five cups of decaf. It's my one addiction that I still allow myself.

I also allowed myself a lot of sweets. But about a month ago, I started to cut back. I got on the scale and said, "Okay, you've had your fun." Now I eat virtually no red meat and watch the fat content in everything.

I never used to eat breakfast, and now I have a bowl of corn flakes with skim milk or maybe a low-fat waffle or two. And for lunch, I'll have a good salad or a veggie sandwich. I wouldn't say that I've gone completely vegetarian—I'll have skinless chicken once a week for my main meal—trying to bring my cholesterol level down. And I take an aspirin every day.

I still don't exercise enough. The only thing that I do is walk, and my wife and I have been talking about that. I need to start on a more active exercise program because one of the things that was prescribed for me was 20 minutes of exercise three times a week, and I have not been doing that faithfully. I work on the fourth floor now, and I do take the stairs maybe a dozen times a day, but I need to do more.

I have a lot of the same problems that a lot of guys do, but I chose to do something about it. And I feel a lot better about myself for getting out of that stressful situation.

I couldn't be happier being out of that rat race. I don't want to be dead in 5 or even 15 years. I finally feel like I've found my mission in life.

A Happy Ending

John Trout, Bethlehem, Pennsylvania

Date of birth: Nov. 17, 1960

Profession: Director of funeral service education, Northampton County Area Community College

Like a lot of couples today, my wife, Kelly, and I decided to work on our marriage and our relationship first and then try to have a family.

Well, once we settled down, we spent the next four years trying to make it happen the old-fashioned way. And when nothing happened, we'd always get the same response from our doctor or friends or relatives: "You're not trying hard enough. Relax. Go away for the weekend. Have a drink before you do it. Go somewhere romantic." All the classic myths about boosting fertility.

But there were other suggestions. I used to wear briefs, but I switched to boxer shorts because that was supposed to keep my sperm cooler. There's a special thing that looks like an athletic supporter that holds either a hot or cold pack. I wore that. We tried sexual positions that you can't even conceive. You've heard the old joke about the turkey baster? I mean, we almost got to the point where we did something like that. We tried anything—regardless of whether it was really out there. But it didn't make any difference. Still no kids.

Then Kelly consulted with her obstetrician/gynecologist, and he recommended that she take her basal body temperature at a certain time of day and chart when she ovulates. (A significant rise in temperature is an indication that ovulation is occurring.) Come to find out, her underactive thyroid, diagnosed many years ago, was influencing her menstrual cycle. Some months she would ovulate, and some months she wouldn't. Some months it was even a different time of the month. Mean-

while, my general practitioner checked me over and couldn't find anything wrong.

Although getting your wife pregnant is a little trickier if she has an irregular menstrual cycle, you ought to be able to get some results within four years. The obstetrician/gynecologist suggested that we see a fertility specialist.

So we went to what's called a reproductive endocrinologist—a fertility specialist—supposedly with extra training in reproductive problems. He ran a number of tests on my wife and reconfirmed the thyroid problem, which we already knew. But really, he said, just keep trying what you're doing—which didn't appease us because we had been trying what we were doing for the last four years.

Fertility Rights

We started going to a local support group called RESOLVE—a national organization—meeting near us once a month for couples who have infertility problems. Many of the people at the meeting were in the same situation—only worse. Many had tried some of the real radical fertility procedures—ones that cost $10,000 to $12,000 a pop and weren't even covered by insurance. A lot of them had second, third and even fourth mortgages; didn't own a car and were still trying to conceive a child. But a couple of them had success stories with a certain doctor. They suggested that we go to him because he also specialized in the male aspect of the equation.

After he saw us, one of the first things he did was send me to a urologist to have a complete checkup—from stem to stern. Among other things, they checked my bladder, my prostate and anything else urological, since that can play a role. I even had a female technician perform a scrotal ultrasound on me. That's what you call an enlightening experience.

You might wonder what this has to do with fertility. But, for example, if you have urine leaking in the wrong place, it can kill sperm—and have a bearing on how fertile you are. They also do a whole semen analysis, detailing the quality and quantity of the sperm. After all that testing, they discovered that I had atrophic testicles, basically the testicles of a five-year-old, and undescended testes.

In a lot of men, atrophic testicles are caused by some kind of sporting accident or a crushing injury of the pelvis, but that never happened to me. I did have mumps though, which, oddly enough, is another cause and enough to give you a low sperm count for life.

So after he reviewed the results, we went back to the fertility specialist, and he said that we could choose between putting my wife on some medicine that would help her produce more eggs and continue trying what I call the old-fashioned way—which, again, would be hit or miss—or create a controlled ovulation cycle in her and use intrauterine insemination (IUI)—artificial insemination. We decided to go with the IUI.

But there was still a lot of work to do for her and for me. Not only was my sperm count low, but they found debris and material in the semen that was unsuitable. It had to be processed—spun and separated and cleansed to get the prime candidates. Even sperm with crooked tails are unacceptable. And that meant that I had to generate more. Much more.

So for months I would go to the doctor's office every four days with a little brown bag and a cup with sperm in it. From the time that it was collected, I had one hour to get it to the doctor's office. When I started I thought that I was going to be the only one doing it. As it turned out, some mornings I had to wait in line because there were six guys in front of me with little paper bags. It's a common problem that may be getting worse. In fact, with the use of pesticides, industrial pollution and everything, I think we might eventually sterilize the human race.

Masturbation was not exactly one of my fortes, and I sure didn't talk publicly about it. But as part of this infertility process, you get to learn how to do it very simply and very clinically. It's somewhat humiliating to start with, but I think about it now and have to laugh. I mean, being told in a doctor's office, "Here's a cup, there's the bathroom, there's a *Playboy* on the back of the toilet—do what comes naturally." And you can hear people talking in the waiting room, and they know what you're doing. But again, I got in the frame of mind that this is the only way that we can conceive a child, and I wasn't going to let it stop us.

Almost Inconceivable

For six months I kept on doing this until they had enough stored in what they call cryo-preserve—basically, freeze-dried sperm—for the procedure. Finally, the day arrived. They took my sperm and injected it into my wife's uterus.

You know what's so funny about it now? We know exactly when conception occurred. There are no ifs, ands or buts like most couples have. We saw an ultrasound of our daughter Madison when she was the size of a grain of sand with a heartbeat. The equipment is that sophisticated. And we went through the same process for our second daughter Kendall, only my wife had some other complications.

Think of it: I could have conceived two children and not even been present for it, but I was, for each procedure. I could have gone out and played golf or gone swimming.

The procedure was expensive but not as expensive as some. For Madison—with ultrasound and medications—it cost about $9,000. With Kendall, my wife had to have some surgery also, so the total was about $22,000.

If you're having this problem, you just have to decide what you want to do—what's important. Do you want to father a child? If you do, then you have to look at all the ways that it can be done. If you're able to do it the natural way, fine. If not, well . . . I'm proof that there are other ways.

And I'd do it again in a heartbeat. I enjoy fatherhood. Our children are everything to us.

Road Map to Health
Your health needs are different at age 50 than they are at age 20. So what you need is a decade-by-decade program that spells out precisely which tests need to be done and which health problems are likely to crop up. Here it is.

The Tests of Time

A Health Plan for Life

The human body requires regular, routine maintenance—just like your car. The only difference is that your car usually comes with a detailed maintenance schedule that tells you when it needs to go into the shop for an oil change or a tune-up or to have the tires rotated. Your body doesn't.

So on the following pages, we've put together simple, concise schedules that take the guesswork out of figuring out which tests you need for every decade of your life.

Here's a brief explanation of all the tests that you will have to have by your seventieth birthday.

Physical examination. The doctor goes over your personal and family health history with you and does a head-to-toe exam, checking out all of your organ systems. The physical does not include blood, urine and other lab tests. That's why they are listed separately.

Blood pressure. This is when the doctor or nurse slips that Velcro tourniquet around your arm, pumps up the pressure and then listens through a stethoscope. It's important to have your blood pressure checked because high blood pressure is a symptomless disease. A normal blood pressure is 120 over 80.

TB skin test. It screens for tuberculosis (TB), which has made a disturbing resurgence in recent years.

Blood and urine tests. They screen for various diseases such as high blood cholesterol, diabetes and kidney disease so that you can catch them before symptoms occur.

Prostate-specific antigen (PSA) test. This is a blood test to determine whether there's something wrong with your prostate. Usually, when something's wrong—such as an infection, enlargement or cancer—your prostate antigen levels rise.

Electrocardiogram. This screens for heart problems.

Rectal exam. The doctor inserts his finger into your anus to check for hemorrhoids, rectal problems and colon and prostate cancer.

Hemoccult. This is done as part of a rectal exam. Some stool is removed and examined for blood, which may mean that there are polyps or colon cancer.

Sigmoidoscopy. A flexible scope is inserted into the rectum and into the colon to diagnose colon cancer at its earliest stages. It also can detect polyps.

Chest x-ray. This should be done yearly in smokers over the age of 45 to help detect lung cancer in an early stage. Usually, lung cancer symptoms don't show up until it's much too late.

Testicular self-exam. You're looking for lumps. For an illustrated explanation of how to perform the exam, see page 95.

Skin self-exam. You're looking for changes in moles, freckles and any unusual skin growths that could be signs of skin cancer.

Eye exam. You go to an ophthalmologist or optometrist to have your eyes checked for vision problems and eye diseases.

Audiogram. This is a test to screen for hearing loss.

Dental checkup. A hygienist will clean your teeth. Then the dentist will check for cavities and other oral problems.

Twenties

As far as your body goes, you are one healthy specimen. You have fewer health worries now than you will have at any time during the rest of your life.

So enjoy these years, but don't think that the way you live today won't have an impact on your future health.

The prime factor that can keep you from seeing your thirtieth birthday is you. Accidents are the leading cause of death for your age group, followed by homicide and suicide. That's all the more reason to not drink and drive, to wear your seat belt and to be a bit more careful out there.

As far as your body is concerned, you do need to watch out for a few cancers that tend to strike younger guys: leukemia, Hodgkin's disease, brain tumors and testicular cancer. "There are certain cancers that occur in younger people and certain cancers that occur in older people, and we just don't really know why," says Sidney J. Winawer, M.D., chief of gastroenterology and nutrition at Memorial Sloan-Kettering Cancer Center in New York City and co-author (with Moshe Shike, M.D., director of clinical nutrition at the center) of *Cancer Free.*

Leukemia is a type of cancer that forms in the blood and blood-forming tissues such as the bone marrow and spleen. Hodgkin's disease is a type of cancer that forms in the lymphatic system, a collection of nodes and vessels that circulates germ-fighting lymph and filters out germs and debris from the body. And brain tumors, as you probably could guess, are a form of cancer that attacks the brain.

None of these cancers are common. But they do occur more often in younger adults and children.

Testicular cancer, however, is one of the most common types of cancer in men ages 20 to 35. The specific cause is unknown, but the cancer is thought to originate with developmental cells in the testes. Testicular cancer is usually detected as a lump on one of the testicles. So it's important to practice monthly self-exams, says Richard Honaker, M.D., of Carrollton, Texas, where he is president of Family Medicine Associates of Texas. See page 95 for an illustrated explanation on how to perform this vital test.

Timelines

- About 5 percent of men start balding in their twenties. If you are one of them, make sure to especially avoid heart disease risk factors such as obesity, smoking and fat-laden foods. Early balding has been linked with an increased risk of heart attack.

- As you make the mental transition from childhood to adulthood, chances are that you're going to be plagued with uncertainties. "How do I know that I'll do okay after college? Will I get a job? Will I get a good job? Will I ever find a woman? Will I ever find the *right* woman?" Those uncertainties are normal.

Putting Yourself to the Test

Physical . . . . .every 3 years	Skin self-exam . . . . .every month
Blood pressure . . . . .every 2 years	Tetanus booster . . . . .once per decade
TB skin test . . . . .every 5 years	Flu shot . . . . .each October
Blood and urine tests . . . .every 3 years	Eye exam . . . . .every 3 years
Electrocardiogram . . . . . .once per decade if high risk	Dental cleaning . . . . . . .every 6 months and exam
Testicular self-exam . . . . .every month	

Thirties

Once you hit your thirties, you need to start monitoring your health a bit more. This is when all the bad things that you did during childhood and early adulthood begin to catch up with you.

Your blood cholesterol and blood pressure levels may begin to climb. That's because all the pizza, potato chips and doughnuts that you survived on in college left fatty deposits on the sides of your arteries, which leaves less room for the blood to flow. Preceded by AIDS and accidents, heart disease becomes the third leading cause of death.

Also, the past 30 years of sun exposure can begin to show up in the form of skin cancer, the most common type of cancer. Skin cancer really hits the scene during your forties, but the average age is getting younger and younger. There are three types of skin cancer: melanoma, basal cell carcinoma and squamous cell carcinoma. Basal and squamous cell carcinoma are very common but seldom deadly. Melanoma, however, spreads quickly and is very deadly.

It's important to start checking your body once a month in search for odd-looking growths that might signal skin cancer. For more information about what to look for, see Moles on page 136. As a general rule, anything that suddenly shows up that wasn't there before should be checked by a health professional.

Another thing to watch out for is stress. It's been linked to just about every health ailment around. And the thirties are by far the most stressful decade of a man's life. It's when you tend to marry, father children, buy a home and really become a responsible adult. You'll be climbing up the ladder at work. And you'll have many financial concerns.

Timelines

• **Unless you keep the muscle that you've built up over the years, your metabolism can slow, making it easier to gain weight.**

• **Though you may not notice it, your ability to hear takes a dip during this decade and will continue to decline until you reach your sixties. Studies show that men experience hearing loss at a rate twice as fast as women.**

• **Your ears start growing, as gravity begins to take its toll on body parts such as your ears and nose. Your earlobes will grow 0.0088 inch each year for the rest of your life. Yes, that's why old men have floppy ears.**

• **Once-flexible joints and cartilage, battered by years of softball and touch football games and general abuse, may ache after extended use.**

Putting Yourself to the Test

Physical	every 3 years	Flu shot	each October
Blood pressure	every 2 years	Eye exam	every 3 years
TB skin test	every 5 years	Glaucoma screening	every 2 years if you have family history of problems; every 3 to 4 years if not
Blood and urine tests	every 3 years		
Electrocardiogram	once if high risk		
Testicular self-exam	every month	Audiogram	only if you have difficulties
Skin self-exam	every month		
Tetanus booster	every 10 years	Dental cleaning and exam	every 6 months

Forties

Maybe you ignored the history of heart disease in your family. Or you ignored your doctor's cautions during your thirties about your rising blood pressure and cholesterol readings. Heck, you probably never even took the time to talk with a doctor about it.

Well, this could very well be the decade that your heart and cardiovascular system make you painfully aware of your neglect. How? For one thing, you may notice that you've become less potent sexually. The fatty goo that's been building up in your arteries all these years usually shuts down the smaller arteries first—namely, those in your penis and even your legs.

Because heart disease becomes more of a health concern during your forties, you need to see a doctor and have your cholesterol tested more frequently than in your younger years. Think of it this way: It may be your last chance to make up for all the time that you never spent with your doctor.

"I don't believe in just sticking your head in the sand and waiting until you are 40 and your artery is 90 percent blocked before you start going to a doctor," says John D. Cantwell, M.D., director of preventive medicine and cardiac rehabilitation at Georgia Baptist Medical Center in Atlanta and chief medical officer of the 1996 Olympic Games. "And I think that you should pick a doctor who is interested in wellness and keeping you healthy."

Timelines

- **Between puberty and this point, your eyesight should have stabilized. But now you become increasingly prone to eye disease as you age. You'll find yourself holding things farther away from your face to read.**

- **You're at an immune high. For once, aging has a positive side. Your immune system is probably working better than it ever has. This will continue into your fifties.**

- **Risk of testicular cancer plummets. Yet another reason to celebrate when you hit the big Four-O: Testicular cancer is extremely rare after forty.**

- **Beware the midlife crisis. This is the time when many men look back and begin to question what they've done with their lives. They realize that the dreams they had in their twenties never materialized. They feel like they didn't succeed. And they become depressed.**

Putting Yourself to the Test

Physical . . . . .every 1 to 2 years
Blood pressure . . . . .every 2 years
Blood and urine tests . . . .every 1 to 2 years
Electrocardiogram . . . . . .every 4 years
Rectal exam . . . . .every year
Chest x-ray . . . . .once a year after age 45 if smoker; chest x-rays for nonsmokers are not recommended
Testicular self-exam . . . . .every month
Skin self-exam . . . . .every month

Tetanus booster . . . . . . .every 10 years
Flu shot . . . . .each October
Eye exam . . . . .every 2 years
Glaucoma screening . . . .every 2 years if you have a family history of problems; every 3 to 4 years if not
Audiogram . . . . .only if you have difficulties
Dental cleaning . . . . . . .every 6 months and exam

Fifties

This is the decade of transition. "For those people who aren't going to make it to the golden years, what they did during the past 50 years is going to catch up with them," says Dr. Honaker.

A surge in testosterone levels causes the prostate to enlarge by as much as 45 percent every ten years for the rest of your life. Once it gets big enough, it will put pressure on the nearby bladder, which can cause urination problems. A quarter of men in their early fifties, half of the men in their sixties and three-quarters of the men in their seventies have enlarged prostates. Male hormones and the aging process also can spur the growth of cancer cells in the prostate, which is why you see the recommendation for annual PSA tests.

Colon cancer also is a concern during this decade. Your colon is lined with tissue that is constantly forming new cells. The new cells rise to the surface and push off the old cells, much the same way that an adult tooth pushes a baby tooth out of the way. But as you age, new cells emerge faster than the body can get rid of the old ones. That forms a bump called a polyp. If not removed, some polyps may turn into cancer in five to ten years.

Timelines

• **If you never snored before, you just might start during this decade. The frequency and intensity of snoring gradually increases with age. That's because tissues in your mouth, nose and throat become less firm, gradually choking off your airway, says John Ruddy, M.D., assistant clinical professor at the National Jewish Center/University of Colorado Health Sciences Center in Denver. If you have always snored, you could eventually develop sleep apnea, which dramatically increases your chances of having a heart attack. Fifty percent of men snore, most of them age 50 and older.**

• **Now here's something to look forward to: Extra unwanted body hair in the ears and nose will really become noticeable during your fifties. Your eyebrow hair will begin to get bushy and seemingly grow straight out instead of sideways.**

• **It's not like it's all downhill here. You've surpassed the uncertainties and worries of your twenties, the stress of your thirties and the depression and midlife crisis of your forties. Now, you'll probably be more at peace with yourself and your life than ever before.**

Putting Yourself to the Test

Physical . . . . .every year	Skin self-exam . . . . .every month
Blood pressure . . . . .every 2 years	Tetanus booster . . . . .every 10 years
Blood and urine tests . . . .every year	Flu shot . . . . .each October
PSA test . . . . .every year	Eye exam . . . . .every 2 years
Electrocardiogram . . . . . .every 3 years	Glaucoma screening . . . .every 2 years if you have family history; every 3 to 4 years if not
Rectal exam . . . . .every year	
Hemoccult . . . . .every year	
Sigmoidoscopy . . . . . . .every 3 to 5 years	Audiogram . . . . .only if you have difficulties
Chest x-ray . . . . .every year if you smoke	
Testicular self-exam . . . . .every month	Dental cleaning . . . . . . .every 6 months and exam

Sixties and Beyond

After age 65, heart disease is the leading cause of death, followed by cancer and stroke.

But even if you survive the big three, you need to pay more attention to mundane ailments such as the flu. As you near 70, your immune system starts to throw in the towel. That's because your thymus gland, the central command of your immune system, has been slowly shrinking throughout your adulthood. It's now one-tenth of the size it was the day you were born.

Compounding the problem is the fact that your white blood cell army simply isn't as abundant or as effective. As a result, diseases that you never had to worry about during your twenties can now become life-threatening.

"By 70 you start to cascade on the down slope. A human body in its tip-top form lives about a century. That is about its viable working duration," says Terry M. Phillips, Ph.D., D.Sc., director of Immunochemistry Labs and professor of medicine at George Washington University Medical Center in Washington, D.C.

Timelines

- **Your hair grows really thin—if, that is, you're one of the lucky few who still has hair. By age 70, 80 percent of men are sporting shiny scalps.**

- **By age 65, upper body strength and muscle tone will decrease by 20 percent, compared to younger adulthood. Fortunately, that atrophy can be offset by a weight-training program.**

- **You can probably stop buying deodorant.** Hormones control your apocrine glands, which are the ones that eventually cause body odor. As you age, you'll begin to smell less as your hormone levels decrease.

- **If you're less active, you're likely to suffer from constipation. Aerobic exercise keeps the bowels moving—and don't forget to keep eating lots of fiber and drinking plenty of water. These steps also will help prevent constipation.**

Once you reach your sixties, you enter a period of growing unrest—literally. You may sleep the same number of hours as when you were 20, but odds are that you no longer sleep straight through the way that you once did, says Dr. John Ruddy of the National Jewish Center/University of Colorado Health Sciences Center.

Putting Yourself to the Test

Physical . . . . .every year	Skin self-exam . . . . .every month
Blood pressure . . . . . . .every 2 years	Tetanus booster . . . . .every 10 years
Blood and urine tests . . . .every year	Flu shot . . . . .each October
PSA test . . . . .every year	Eye exam . . . . .every 1 to 2 years
Electrocardiogram . . . . . .every 3 years	Glaucoma screening . . . .every 2 years if you have family history; every 3 to 4 years if not
Rectal exam . . . . .every year	
Hemoccult . . . . .every year	
Sigmoidoscopy . . . . . . .every 3 to 5 years	Audiogram . . . . .every 2 to 3 years
Chest x-ray . . . . .every year if you smoke	Dental cleaning . . . . . . .every 6 months and exam
Testicular self-exam . . . . .every month	

Index

Note: Underscored page references indicate boxed text or illustrations. **Boldface** references indicate primary discussion of topic.

A

A and D ointment, 51
Accidents, 16–17, 17
Accutane, 127
Achilles tendons, 102
Acne, **126–27**, 127
Acupressure, 47, 50, 53, 54, 80, 117
Acyclovir, 133
Adrenaline, 51, 68
Afrin, 50
Agility, improving, 102
Air cast, 101
Air filter, breathing problems and, 63
Alcohol
    bruising and, 132
    cluster headaches and, 48
    forgetfulness and, 41
    hangover from, 45
    heartburn and, 75–76
    in heart disease prevention, 66, 68
    impotence and, 84–85
    incontinence and, 78
    nausea from, 79
    nosebleed and, 51
    snoring and, 55
    urination problems and, 98
Allergens, 10, 52, 62–63
Allergies, **10–11**, 39, 52, 54, 62, 137
Allergy Control Products, 63
Alpha hydroxy acids, 126–27
Amino acid imbalance, 34
Anal ailments, **70**
Androderm, 90

Angina, 64
Ankle pain, **100–102**
Antacids, 65, 72–73, 76
Antibacterial ointment, 133
Antibodies, allergies and, 10
Antidepressants, 72, 88
Antigens, 4
Antihistamines, 11, 53–54, 138
Antioxidants, 113
Antiperspirants, 131
Anti-wart preparations, 140
Aphrodisiacs, 84–85
Apocrine glands, 130, 163
Arches, ankle pain and, 102, 114
Arm pain, **103**
Arnica, 107, 132
Arousal, 91
Arthritis, 109, 111, 112–13
Aspirin, 40, 44, 59, 65, 76, 80, 138
Asthma, 62–63
Athlete's foot, **128–29**
Attitude, immune system and, 9
Audiogram, 158
Aveeno, 138

B

Back pain, **104–8**
Bacteria, 4–5, 52, 73, 74, 126, 131
Bad breath, **32**
Baking soda, rashes and, 137–38
Baldness, **42–43**, 43, 159, 163
Balloon carpal tunnel-plasty, 124
Bananas, potassium replacement and, 73
Basis soap, 138
Bathing, 135, 138
B cells, 7–8
Beamon, Bob, **148–49**
Beano, 74
Belching, **71**
Benadryl, 34, 54, 80, 138
Benign prostatic hyperplasia (BPH), 96–97
Benzoyl peroxide, 126

Beta-carotene, 113
Bioflavonoids, 60
Bladder problems, 77–78, 96–98
Bleeding gums, **33**
Bleeding problems, 27, 33, 70
Blood pressure, 41, 122
Blood pressure test, 158
Blood test, 29, 158
Blowing nose, 51, 53
Body, listening to, **2–3**, 3, 45
Body odor, **130–31**, 163
Body strength, decreasing, 163
Boron intake, 41
Boxer shorts, fertility and, 93
BPH, 96–97
Brace, elbow, 110
Bread, 66
Breathing problems, 26–27, 56, **62–63**
Breathing techniques, 103
Breath odor, **32**
Broken nose, 51
Bronchitis, 62
Bronchodilator, 62
Bruises, 101, **132**
Brushing teeth, 32–33
Brushing test, 32–33
Bruxism, 49
Bupropion hydrochloride, 89
Bursitis, 111, 120
B vitamins, 39, 65–66

C

Caffeine
    diarrhea and avoiding, 73
    hay fever and, 54
    heartbeat irregularities and avoiding, 68
    heartburn and avoiding, 75–76
    incontinence and, 78
    tension-type headaches and avoiding, 44
    urination problems and avoiding, 98
Calcium, 93
Calories, metabolism and, 13

Cancer
    bone marrow, 159
    colon, 70, 162
    growths leading to, 28
    personal experience with,
        152–53
    preventing, 15–17
    prostate, 97
    semen problems and, 92
    skin, 136
    testicular, 94, 159, <u>161</u>
Candy, sore throat and hard, 57
Canker sores, **34**
Car accidents, <u>16–17</u>
Carbonated drinks, 59, 71
Cardiovascular disease, 82
Cardura, 98
Carpal tunnel syndrome, 103,
    109, 122–23
Cartilage, 111
Casein, 72
Cavities, 59
Cereals, 66
Cervical neck collar, 118
Cetaphil lotion, 126
Chamomile, 138
Chapped lips, **35**
Chemoreceptor trigger zone, <u>80</u>
Chest pain, 26, **64–66**
Chest x-ray, 158
Chiggers, 137
Chiropractors, 106
Chlamydia, 97
Cholesterol, 11, 29, 37, 66, 85–86
Cholesterol screening, 66
Cigarette smoking
    back pain and avoiding,
        107–8
    carpal tunnel syndrome and
        avoiding, 122
    cluster headaches and avoid-
        ing, 48
    heart disease and avoiding, 66
    impotence and avoiding, 85
    quitting, <u>14–15</u>
    snoring and avoiding, 56
Cinnamon, 41

Citrucel, 72
Clean & Clear acne product, 126
Clove, oil of, 59
Cluster headaches, **48**
Coal tar shampoo, 134
Cocaine, 68
Codeine, 36, 138
Coffee, 54, 63, 75–76, 78. *See
    also Caffeine*
Coke, defizzed, 79
Cold, common, **52–54**
Cold compresses, 135, 137
Cold foods, 68
Cold sores, **133**
Collagen injection, 78
Combing hair, 43
Compresses, cool, 40
Condom, 97
Congestion, nasal, 52–53
Conover, Mark, **146–47**
Constipation, 70, **72**, 78, <u>163</u>
Cortisone cream, 137
Coughing, **36**, 62
Cough suppressants, 36
Counseling, 68, 90
Cramps, **117**
Cutting/styling hair, 43
Cycling, 97, 112

D

Dairy Ease, 74
Dairy products, 72–74
Dandruff, **134**
Decongestants, 38, 50, 53, 55, 68
Deer hoof's gland, odors and,
    <u>129</u>
Dehydration, 117
Dental checkup, 158
Dental problems. *See specific
    types*
Dentists, <u>19</u>, 49
Deodorants, 131
Depression, 88, 90
Dextromethorphan, 36
Diabetes, 28, 87, 93, 122
Dial soap, 131

Diarrhea, 70, **73**
Diet
    acne and, 127
    allergies and, 11
    bad breath and, 32
    bleeding gums and, 33
    canker sores and, 34
    diarrhea and, 73
    heartbeat irregularities and, 68
    immune system and, 8
    impotence and, 82
    jaw pain and, 49
    migraine headaches and,
        46–47
    nausea/vomiting and, 79–80
    runny/stuffy nose and, 53
    tension headaches and, 45
    unhealthy, 12–13
    urination problems and, 98
Dieting, 13
Digestive problems, **70–80**. *See
    also specific types*
Dimethyl phythalate, 138
Diphenhydramine, 36, 54, 138
Dizziness, 2, 27, **37**
DNA, 5, 16
Doctors, **18–30**
    abbreviations used by, <u>29</u>
    cooperating with, 22–23
    interviewing techniques for,
        20–22
    issues in selecting, 18–20
    male view of visiting, <u>22–23</u>
    money- and time-saving tips
        about, <u>20–21</u>
    physical exams by, 28–30
    second opinions and, 30
    standing up for self and,
        24–25
    symptoms requiring visit to,
        26–28
    traveling and, <u>25</u>
    visits to, 18
Dove soap, 138
Doxazosin, 98
Dracunculus medinensis, <u>6–7</u>
Dramamine, 79, <u>80</u>

Drugs. *See* Prescription drugs; *specific types*
Dry skin, 135
Duofilm, 140
Duoplant Gel, 140
Duration decongestant spray, 50
Dvorak, Joe, **152–53**
Dysentery, 73

E

Ear drops, 38
Earlobes, growth of, 160
Ear pain, **38**
Ear wax, removing, 38
Eccrine glands, 130
Echinacea, 58
Eczema, 128
Egg white, 126
Ejaculate, 93
Elbow pain, **109–10**
Electrocardiogram, 158
Emetrol, 79
Emotional support, 89
Emphysema, 62
Endorphins, 47
Eosinophils, 10
Epididymis, 94
Erections, 83, 87, 91. *See also*
    Impotence
Essential fatty acids, 39
Estrogen, 12, 92
Exercise
    aerobic, 14, 108, 163
    anaerobic, 14
    asthma from, 62
    in cold, 62
    eating before, 76
    effects of, on
        breathing problems, 62–63
        cluster headaches, 48
        constipation, 72
        health, 13–14
        immune system, 9
        impotence, 82, 86
    for eyes, 60

indoor, 63
for preventing
    back pain, 106–7, 106, 108
    heart attack, 66
sudden vs. steady, 68
swimming, 63
switch-hitting in, 105
time of day for, best, 63
for treating
    ankle pain, 101
    elbow pain, 110
    knee pain, 112–13
    leg pain, 115
    neck pain, 119, 119
    shoulder pain, 121
    wrist pain, 123, 124
weight-lifting belt and, 106
Eyebrow hair, 139
Eye discomfort, **39**
Eye disease, 161
Eye exam, 158

F

Fat intake, 13, 66, 76
Fatty acids, 134–35
Fear, **150–51**
Fertility, personal experience
    about, 156–57
Fever, 5, 28, **40**
Fiber, 13, 66, 70, 72, 163
Fiber supplements, 72–73
Filter, breathing problems and, 63
Fish, 11, 39
Flatulence, **74**
Flaxseed, 39, 66
Flexibility, 117
Flossing teeth, 32–33, 59
Fluid intake
    anal ailments and, 70
    chapped lips and, 35
    constipation and, 72, 163
    fever and, 40
    incontinence and, 78
    runny/stuffy nose and, 53
    sore throat and, 57

Flu shot, 30
Folate, 65–66
Folic acid, 65–66
Food allergies, 11, 62
Food Guide Pyramid, 13
Foods. *See* Diet; *specific types*
Foot alignment, 108
Forgetfulness, **41**
Fracture, ankle, 101–2
Fruits, 13, 41, 66, 72
Fungi, 5, 70, 128

G

Garlic, 57–58, 85–86, 129
Gas, intestinal, 71, 74
Gastroesophageal reflux, 36
Gas-X, 71
Gatorade, 73, 76
Germs, **4–9**, 5
Ginger, 57–58, 79
Ginkgo, 41
Glucosamine sulfate, 39
Glutathiones, 60
Glycolic acid peels, 127
Goldenseal, 58
Golfer's elbow, 109
Gonorrhea, 97
Gout, 109
Grains, 66
Grinding teeth, 49
Grover's disease, 137
Guaifensin, 36
Guinea worms, 6–7
Gum chewing
    bad breath and, 32
    belching and avoiding, 71
    diarrhea and avoiding, 73
    heartburn and, 75
    tooth decay and, 59

H

Hair loss, 42–43, 43, 159, 163
Hair pieces, 43
Hair products, 134
Hair transplant surgery, 42–43

Halitosis, **32**
Hangovers, <u>45</u>
Harper, Charles M., **142–43**
Hay fever, 54
HDL cholesterol, 12, 29, 66
Headaches, **44–48**, <u>47</u>
Head & Shoulders shampoo, 134
Health maintenance, **12–17,
    158–63**
  in fifties, 162, <u>162</u>
  in forties, 161, <u>161</u>
  in sixties and beyond, 163,
      <u>163</u>
  suggestions for, 12–17, <u>14–15,
      16–17</u>
  tests, 158
  in thirties, 160, <u>160</u>
  in twenties, 159, <u>159</u>
Health maintenance organization
    (HMO), 30
Health problems. *See also
    specific types*
  lingering, 28
  personal experiences with,
      142–57
  shoes and, 101–2, 116, 131
  sleep and, 9, 41, 45, <u>47</u>,
      55–56
Healthy Scalp shampoo, 134
Heart attack, 64–66
Heartbeat irregularities, **67–68**
Heartburn, 65, 71, **75–76**, <u>76</u>
Heart disease risk, 42
Heart palpitations, 67–68
Heart problems, **62–68**. *See also
    specific types*
Heat rash, 137
Heat treatment, 101, 118, 121
Hemoccult, 158
Hemorrhoids, 70
Heredity
  acne and, 126
  body hair and, 139
  hair loss and, 42
  heart disease risk and, 65
  melanomas and, 136

Herpesviruses, 133
High blood pressure, 122
Histamine, 39, 53
Hives, 137–38
HMO, 30
Hodgkin's disease, 159
Honey potion, 36, 57
Hormones, 126, 130, 162, <u>163</u>.
    See also specific types
Hrabar, Greg, **150–51**
Humidifiers, stuffy nose and, 52
Hygiene, 8–9, 70, 133
Hyperhidrosis, 130
Hytrin, 98

I

Ibuprofen, 44, 59, 80, 109, 138
Ice treatment for
  anal ailments, 70
  back pain, 105
  jaw pain, 49
  leg pain, 115
  neck pain, 118
  nosebleed, 50, <u>51</u>
  rashes, 137
  tension-type headache, 44
  toothache, 59
  wrist pain, 123
Imitrex, 47
Immune system, **4–9**
  allergens and, 10
  attitude and, 9
  enhancing, 8–9
  in forties, <u>161</u>
  garlic and, 58
  germs affecting, 4–9, <u>5</u>
  healing power and, 27
  immunity and, 7–9
  in sixties and beyond, 163
  stress and, 9
Immunizations, 8, <u>30</u>
Immunotherapy, 11, 78, <u>83</u>,
    86–87
Impotence, **82–87**
  causes of, 82–84
  incidence of, 82

low sex drive and, 88
  preventing, 84–87
  as symptom of health
      problem, 27–28
Incontinence, **77–78**, 98
Inderal, 47
Infection, 58
Infertility, **156–57**
Inflammation, 64
Interstitial cystitis, 97
Isotretinoin, 127
Itchy skin, **135**

J

Jaw pain, **49**
Jock itch, **128–29**

K

Kaopectate, 34
Kenalog, 34
Ketone, <u>129</u>
Kidney dysfunction, 122
Kneecap pain, 112, <u>114</u>
Knee pain, **111–14**, <u>114</u>

L

Lacriminal gland, 39
Lactaid, 74
Lactase, 74
Lactose intolerance, 73
LDL cholesterol, 12, 29, 66
Lead, 92
Leg pain, **115–16**
Lesions, precancerous, 35
Leukemia, 159
Lever 2000 soap, 131
Libido, low, 88–90
Ligaments, 100, 111, 120
Lighting, migraines and, 47
Lip balm, 35
Lipid profile, 29
Localized neurodermis, 135
Longevity, 12
Low sex drive, **88–90**, <u>90</u>

Lozenges, 57
Lubricating creams, nose, 51
Lumbar supports, 107
Lung problems, **62–63**. *See also specific types*
Lymph nodes, 58
Lysine tablets, 34

M

Magnesium, 46, 63, 67–68
Massage, 44–45, 117–18
Melanin, 35
Melanoma, 136
Memory loss, **41**
Ménière's disease, 37
Menthol, 36
Mentholatum, 51
Messages, body, **2–3**, 3, 45
Mesylate, 98
Metabolism, 160
Metamucil, 72
MG217 shampoo, 134
Miconazole, 128
Midlife crisis, 161
Migraine headaches, 44, **46–47**, 47
Miliaria, 137
Milk, 11, 73, 76, 93
Minerals, 67–68. *See also specific types*
Minoxidil, 43
Moisturizers, 127, 135
Moles, **136**
Monosodium glutamate (MSG), 45
Mortality rates, 12, 15
Motion sickness, 80
MSG, 45
Muscle cramps, **117**
Muscle tone, decreasing, 163
Mylanta Gas Relief, 71

N

Nasal sprays, 50, 53, 55
Nasal strips, 53

Nausea, **79–80**
Neck pain, **118–19**
Neo-Synephrine, 50
Neutrogena shampoo, 134
Nicotine, 66. *See also* Cigarette smoking
Nirschl Counter Force brace, 110
Nonsteroidal anti-inflammatory drug (NSAID), 105, 138
Nosebleed, **50–51**, 53
NSAID, 105, 138

O

Oatmeal bath, 138
Obesity, 70. *See also* Overweight
Odor, body, **130–31**, 163
Off! Skintastic, 138
Olajidé, Michael, Jr., **144–45**
Olive oil, 134
Orange juice, 93, 112–13
Orthotics, 102, 114
Osteoarthritis, 112
Overweight, 63, 70, 75, 112, 114. *See also* Weight loss
Oxygen, cluster headaches and, 48

P

Painkillers, 44, 72. *See also specific types*
P&S Shampoo, 134
Parasites, 5–6
Patellofemoral pain, 112, 114
Penile implant, 86–87
Penile warts, 140
Peppermint, 76
Pepto-Bismol, 80
Phentolamine mesylate, 83
Phlegm, 36
Phobias, **150–51**
Physical examination, 158
Physical therapists, 121
Pinworms, 70

Pizza burn, 33
Plantar warts, 140
Plaque, 33, 82
Poison ivy/oak/sumac, 138
Pollen, 10, 39, 62–63
Polyps, 28, 162
Polysporin, 133
Popcorn-kernel syndrome, 33
Posture, good, 119
Potassium, 46, 67–68
Premature ejaculation, 88, **91**
Prescription drugs
  abbreviations for, 29
  effects of, on
    constipation, 72
    heartburn, 76
    impotence, 83
    incontinence, 78
    low sex drive, 88
    money-saving tips, 27
  for treating
    cold sores, 133
    urination problems, 98
Pressure treatments, 50, 51, 54
Pressurized mask, snoring and, 56
Priapism, 83
Prickly heat, 137
Progesterone, 12
Propranolol, 47
Prostaglandin, 82
Prostaglandin E_1, 83, 86–87
Prostate gland, 77–78, 97, 162
Prostate-specific antigen (PSA), 29, 158, 162
Prostatitis, 97
Protein products, 74
PSA, 29, 158, 162
Pseudoephedrine, 38
Psoriasis, 134
Pus, 5, 38

R

Rashes, 128, **137–38**
Rectal exam, 28–29, 158
Reflexes, 113–14

Regitine, <u>83</u>
Relaxation treatment, 45, <u>51</u>, 71, 84, 91
Repetitive-motion injuries, 103, 109
Rest, 65, 103, 105, 121
Rest, ice, compression and elevation (RICE) treatment, 100–101, 112
Retainers, snoring and, 56
Retin-A, 127
Reye's syndrome, 40
RICE treatment, 100–101, 112
Rogaine, 43
Rosemary, 52
Rotator cuff, 120
Runner's trots, 73
Runny/stuffy nose, **52–53**

S

Safeguard soap, 131
Salicylic acid, 126, 134, 140
Saliva production, 32, 59, 75
Salt intake, reducing, 37
Salt-water rinse, 34, 57, 128
Saw palmetto berry, 97
Scents, <u>131</u>
Second opinions, 30
Selenium sulfide, 134
Selsun Blue shampoo, 134
Semen problems, **92–93**
Serotonin, 46
Sex problems, **82–98**. *See also specific types*
Sexually transmitted disease (STD), 97
Shampoos, 134
Shaving hair, 139
Shinsplints, 116, <u>116</u>
Shoes, health problems and, 101–2, 116, 131
Shortness of breath, 26–27
Shoulder pain, **120–21**
Sigmoidoscopy, 28–29, 158
Simethicone, 71

Sitting position, back problems and, 105
Skin problems, **126–40**. *See also specific types*
Skin self-exam, 158
Skin tests, 11
Sleep, health problems and, 9, 41, 45, <u>47</u>, 55–56
Sleep apnea, <u>56</u>, <u>162</u>
Sleep positions, 55, 75, 120–21, 123
Slurping, avoiding, 71
Snacking, avoiding, 55
Sneezing, 8, **54**
Snoring, **55–56**, <u>162</u>
Soap, 131, 135, 138
Soda, 59, 71
Sorbitol, 71, 73–74
Sore throat, **57**
Sperm count, 92–93
SPF, 35, 132, 136
Sphincter muscles, 77–78
Spicy foods, 34, 53, 59, 68, 75
Splints, wrist, 123
Sports medicine doctors, 111
Sprained ankle, 100
STD, 97
Steak, treating bruises with, 132
Steam treatment, 53
Steroid sprays, 11
Stomach acid, **75–76**
Stomach and digestive system problems, **70–80**. *See also specific types*
Stress, 9, 14–15, 68
Stretching, 44, 108, 110, 113, 115, 124
Sudafed, 78
Sugar, 57
Sumatriptan, 47
Sunburn, 35
Sunglasses, sneezing and, 54
Sun protection factor (SPF), 35, 132, 136
Support groups, 68
Surgical treatments, 42–43, 56, <u>86–87</u>, 98, 114, <u>124</u>

Sweat, 130–31, 137
Swelling, <u>5</u>
Swimming, 63
Swollen glands, **58**

T

Tai chi, improved agility and, 37
Tartar, 33
TB skin test, 158
T cells, 7–8
Tegrin shampoo, 134
Temporomandibular disorder (TMD), 49
Tendinitis, 120
Tendons, 101, 102, 109, 120
Tennis elbow, 109–10
TENS unit, 106
Testicular exam, 29–30, <u>95</u>, 158
Testicular injuries, 92
Testicular lumps, **94–95**
Testosterone, 42, 87–88, 139
Testosterone transdermal system, 90
Tetrazosin hydrochloride, 98
Theophylline, 63
Thirst, increased, 28
Thoracic outlet syndrome, 103
Tissues, vs. handkerchiefs, 8
TMD, 49
Toilet habits, 72
Toilet paper, 70
Toothache, **59**
Tooth decay, <u>76</u>
Toothpastes, 35
Transcutaneous electrical nerve stimulator (TENS) unit, 106
Trapezius muscles, 119
Tretinoin, 127
Triamcinolone acetonide, 34
Trout, John, **156–57**
Tuck pads, 70
Type A personalities, 48

U

Ulcer, 80
Ulnar nerve compression, 109
Underwear, fertility and, 93
Unwanted hair growth, **139**, 162
Urination problems, **96–98**, 98
Urine test, 29, 158

V

Vaccinations, 8
Vacuum therapy, 87
Vegetables, 13, 41, 60, 66, 72
Vent brush, 43
Vics VapoRub, 51
Vinegar, white, 38
Viruses, 5, 52, 140
Vision problems, **60**
Vitamin A, 60
Vitamin B$_6$, 123–24

Vitamin C, 93, 112–13
Vitamin E, 65, 112–13
Vitamin K cream, 132
Vitamins, 9. *See also specific types*
Vomiting, **79–80**

W

Walker, Charlie, **154–55**
Walking, 112–13
Walking backward, 114
Warm-ups, 121
Wart-Off, 140
Warts, **140**
Washing hair, 43, 134
Weight gain, 160
Weight loss, 55–56, 63, 70, 75, 107. *See also* Overweight
Wellbutrin, 89
Wheezing, 62
Whistling, snoring and, 55

White blood cells, 40, 58, 163
Wine, 41, 66
Wraps, bandage, 102
Wrinkles, 126
Wrist pain, **122–24**

X

X-rays, 101–2, 158
X-Seb shampoo, 134

Y

Yeasts, 134
Yohimbine, 84–85, 89

Z

Zinc, 86, 93, 97–98
Zincon shampoo, 134
Zinc pyrithione, 134
Zovirax, 13